Unusual Cases in Peritoneal Surface Malignancies

Emel Canbay

Editor

Unusual Cases in Peritoneal Surface Malignancies

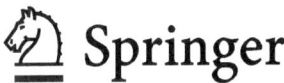 Springer

Editor
Emel Canbay
Peritoneal Dissemination Treatment
Istanbul
Turkey

ISBN 978-3-319-51522-9   ISBN 978-3-319-51523-6   (eBook)
DOI 10.1007/978-3-319-51523-6

Library of Congress Control Number: 2017933480

Printed on acid-free paper

This Springer imprint is published by Springer Nature
The registered company is Springer International Publishing AG
The registered company address is: Gewerbestrasse 11, 6330 Cham, Switzerland

Preface

Peritonectomy Procedures have been described by the inspiring leader in the field, Paul H. Sugarbaker. Cytoreductive Surgery with Heated Intraoperative Intraperitoneal Chemotherapy and Intraperitoneal Chemotherapy Applications have gradually evolved over the past three decades to manage peritoneal malignancies. These procedures were extensively discussed in our first book entitled "Peritoneal Surface Malignancies: A Curative Approach" published in 2015 by Springer.

Following my extensive clinical fellowships with Yutaka Yonemura and Paul H. Sugarbaker, the approach in Turkey was established in which surgical approaches and chemotherapy applications are used. These procedures inspired my surgical brain and enthused me to establish the Peritoneal Surface Malignancy Center in Turkey as the basis of my life interest.

The initial descriptions in the management of peritoneal surface malignancies involve the treatment of epithelial appendiceal malignancies, peritoneal metastases of colorectal cancer, gastric cancer, and ovarian cancer, and primary peritoneal malignancies as peritoneal mesothelioma and peritoneal serous carcinomas.

Unusual cases with Peritoneal Surface Malignancies are challenging and clinical situations for these are often seen in international centers. Therefore, this book was written to unite the worldwide effort in this field.

The reader will learn about the management approaches for cases with peritoneal surface malignancies that are rarely seen. The Editor expresses deep gratitude to all authors of the book, Mr. Andre Tournois and Ms. Geetha Dhandapani and Evgenia Koutsouki from Springer, for their enormous efforts to make this work come true. This book seeks to promote the extension of the comprehensive approaches to unusual cases with peritoneal surface malignancies.

The proper and increased use of these modalities by the multidisciplinary team and the prompt referral of these patients for definitive management are the major goals of all the authors in this book.

Our international leaders Paul H. Sugarbaker and Yutaka Yonemura and all others have suffered too much to establish that peritoneal metastasis can be prevented and eliminated in cases with intraabdominal malignancies and gynecologic malignancies. This is the time to increase the efforts to extend this knowledge to a younger generation of surgeons and medical oncologists and related clinical disciplins in all over the world.

Peritoneal Malignancy is a new frontier and this book discusses the treatment strategies for unusual cases. We all hope the reader will find this book useful. We publish this volume as the first series of contributions and we aim to update this periodically. We look forward to extend the international participation to this effort.

Istanbul, Turkey   Emel Canbay

Contents

Chapter 1
Peritoneal Metastasis from Small Bowel Adenocarcinoma Associated with Crohn's Disease

Emel Canbay

1.1 Introduction

Crohn's disease (CD) is a clinical condition characterized by inflammation of the intestines that may involve the entire thickness of the intestinal walls. CD most often involves the small intestine and colon. Over the past decades, intestinal adenocarcinoma has been recognized as a complication of CD. The management of patients with peritoneal metastasis (PM) of small bowel adenocarcinoma (SBA) associated with Crohn's disease (CD) has not been defined yet. This report will be structured as a case report of PM of SBA associated with CD.

From this data, other peritoneal surface oncology centers may wish to offer CRS and HIPEC to patients with similar features at early stages of this disease.

1.2 Small Bowel Adenocarcinoma Associated with CD

Small bowel adenocarcinoma (SBA) has been found to be associated with Crohn's disease (CD). In 1956, SBA associated with CD has been reported by Ginzburg for the first time [1]. Since then, there are numerous studies that have published the occurrence of small bowel carcinoma developed from CD.

The relative risk of developing small bowel carcinoma in patients with CD was 28.37 in 9,642 patients [2]. The mean duration of CD before the onset of adenocarcinoma was 9 (range 0.8–41) years [2]. Risk factors for small bowel are listed in Table 1.1.

E. Canbay, MD, PhD
Center for Peritoneal Surface Oncology, NPO HIPEC Istanbul,
Guzelbahce Sokak No:15, Istanbul, Turkey
e-mail: drecanbay@gmail.com

© Springer International Publishing AG 2017
E. Canbay (ed.), *Unusual Cases in Peritoneal Surface Malignancies*,
DOI 10.1007/978-3-319-51523-6_1

1

Table 1.1 Risk factors for developing small bowel carcinoma in patients with CD

Crohn's related risk factors for small bowel adenocarcinoma
Long duration of CD
Area of CD inflammation
Jejunal CD
Strictures
Fistula
Bypassed segment
CD medications
Young age
Male gender
Tobacco-alcohol-diet

The most common clinical presentation of SBA associated with CD is obstruction with nausea, vomiting, and abdominal pain. Other presentations are hemorrhage, fistula, and perforation [3–4]. These symptoms are commonly seen in CD's exacerbation, and it is almost always difficult to differentiate small bowel adenocarcinoma from those of the CD's activation. Majority of the patients with SBA associated with CD are diagnosed at the time of operation or postoperatively and only less than 5% cases are diagnosed preoperatively [3]. Two indicators of the malignancy in patients with CD are exacerbation of the symptoms after long periods of the quiescence and small bowel obstruction refractory to medical treatments [4]. Therefore, it is important to consider surgical assessment of patients with long-standing symptomatic CD who failed to respond to conservative treatments.

The age of diagnosis of SBA associated with CD is 45–55 years [3, 4]. Even though de novo SBA are seen all along the small intestine, SBA associated with CD is almost located within the inflamed areas of the ileum [4–6].

Diagnosis of SBA associated with CD is often challenging. Imaging techniques may miss lesions smaller than 0.5 cm and not be able to distinguish the affected areas from severe CD.

SBA staging can be 47% accurate with computed tomography (CT); however sensitivity is very low in the presence of CD [7]. CT exposes patients to radiation, and magnetic resonance (MR) imaging is not, but MRI takes much longer time and cost is expensive [8]. Enteroclysis is invasive and training is required for exact diagnosis of SBA associated with CD [9]. Positron emission tomography (PET) is used within limits in the diagnosis of SBA associated with CD due to chronic inflammation [10]. Multiphasic dynamic studies may have the potential to improve the diagnostic capacity of multidetector CT for SBA [11].

SBA associated with CD are mainly adenocarcinoma, very rare signet ring cell carcinoma [12].

The prognosis of SBA associated with CD has been reported to be poorer than the de novo small bowel carcinoma [13].

To date, there is no any report regarding the incidence and prognosis as well as management of peritoneal metastasis (PM) from SBA associated with CD. Here, we report our case of a patient with PM from SBA associated with CD who had a limited survival.

1.3   Case Report

A 51-year-old male patient with a history of Crohn's disease for 30 years developed intestinal obstruction in June 2014. Through a midline incision, he underwent resection of the terminal ileum. Pathological investigations revealed adenocarcinoma of the ileum developed from CD. He underwent a strictureplasty and small bowel resections 10 years ago due to CD. In July 2014, he developed an intestinal obstruction and returned back to the operating room for right hemicolectomy and segmental small bowel resection. The patient had five cycles of adjuvant systemic chemotherapy with FOLFOX, and he developed peritoneal metastasis after systemic chemotherapy. Then, six cycles of FOLFIRI + bevacizumab were given. His PET scan shows the peritoneal metastasis due to seeding from his previous operations.

Positron emission tomography (PET), computerized tomography (CT), PET-CT, and computerized axial tomography (CAT) scans of the patient with PM from SBA associated CD are given in Figs. 1.1, 1.2, 1.3, 1.4, 1.5, and 1.6. The patient developed partial intestinal obstruction in December 2015. The patient was presented to the American Society of Peritoneal Surface Malignancy multidisciplinary team via

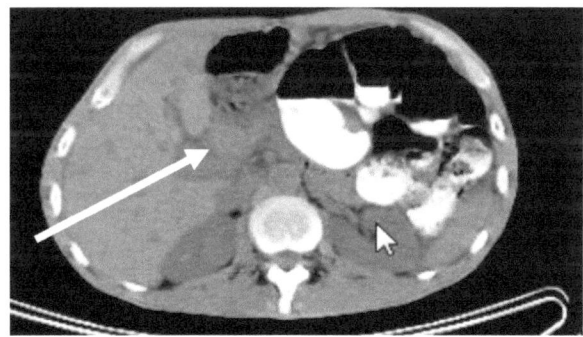

Fig. 1.1 The mass in the anterior abdominal wall in axial CT scan. *Arrow* shows the intra-abdominal metastatic mass in patients with SBA associated with CD

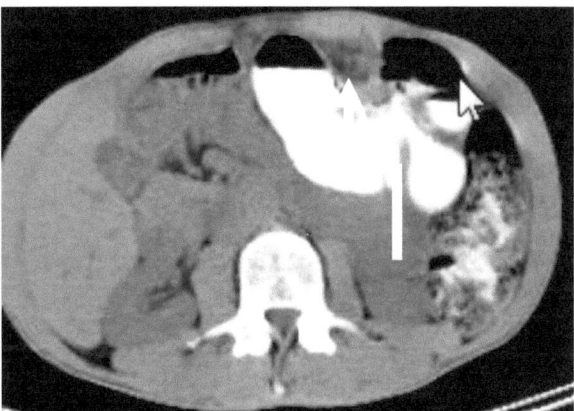

Fig. 1.2 The mass in the anterior abdominal wall in axial CT scan. *Arrow* indicates the metastatic tumor in patients with SBA associated with CD

the Internet. Only a limited outcome has been introduced from all over the world. They all concluded that the management of PM from SBA associated with CD is poor. His perioperative findings revealed that he had a recurrence in the ileo-transversostomy site and with extensive peritoneal metastasis (Figs. 1.7, 1.8, and

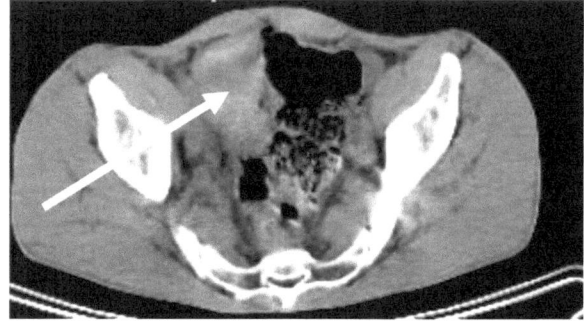

Fig. 1.3 The mass in the lower anterior abdominal wall in axial CT view. *Arrow* indicates the metastatic abdominal mass in patients with small bowel adenocarcinoma (SBA) associated with Crohn's disease (CD)

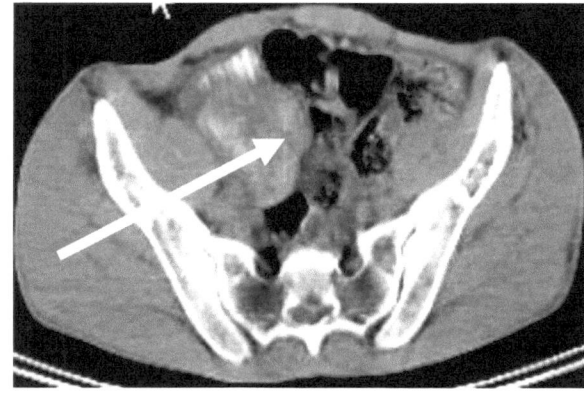

Fig. 1.4 The mass in the lower anterior abdominal wall in axial CT view. *Arrow* indicates the metastatic abdominal mass in patients with small bowel adenocarcinoma (SBA) associated with Crohn's disease (CD)

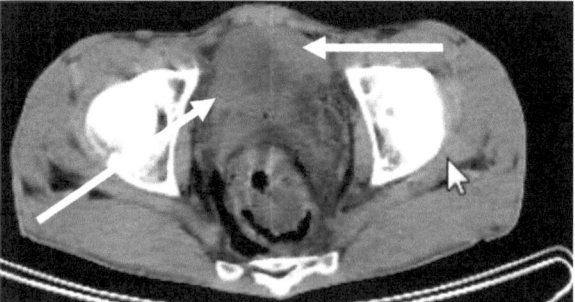

Fig. 1.5 The masses in the lower anterior abdominal wall in axial CT view. *Arrows* indicate the metastatic abdominal mass in patients with SBA associated with CD

1.9). His perioperative PCI score was 30. He underwent a cytoreductive surgery and terminal ileostomy and hyperthermic intraoperative intraperitoneal chemotherapy. The small bowel was around 120 cm and had multiple metastatic nodules after the

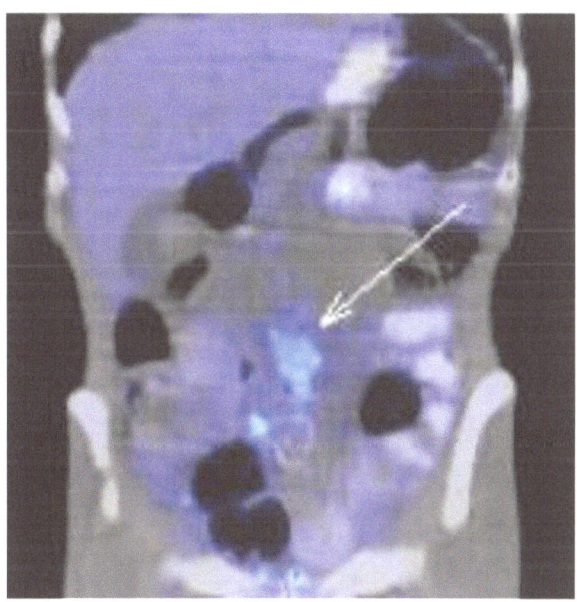

Fig. 1.6 A PET-CT scan of the peritoneal metastasis of the patients with small bowel adenocarcinoma associated with Crohn's disease. *Arrow* indicates the peritoneal nodules

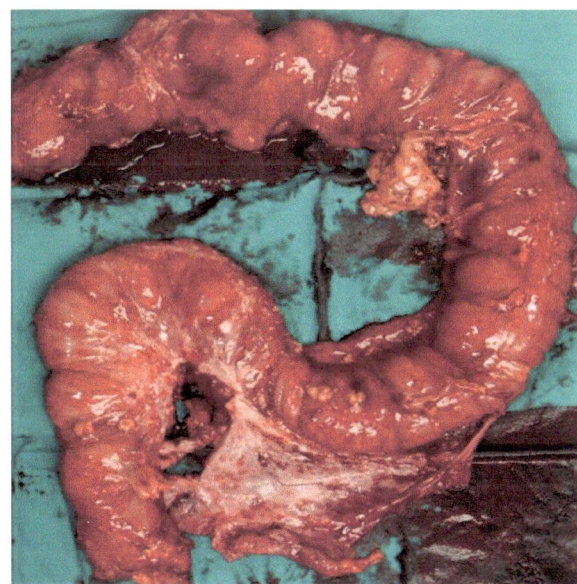

Fig. 1.7 The anastomotic ileo-transversostomy site, transvers colon, left colon and sigmoid colon, upper rectum, and pelvic peritoneum are heavily involved with metastatic nodules

Fig. 1.8 Anastomotic site recurrence is detected preoperatively

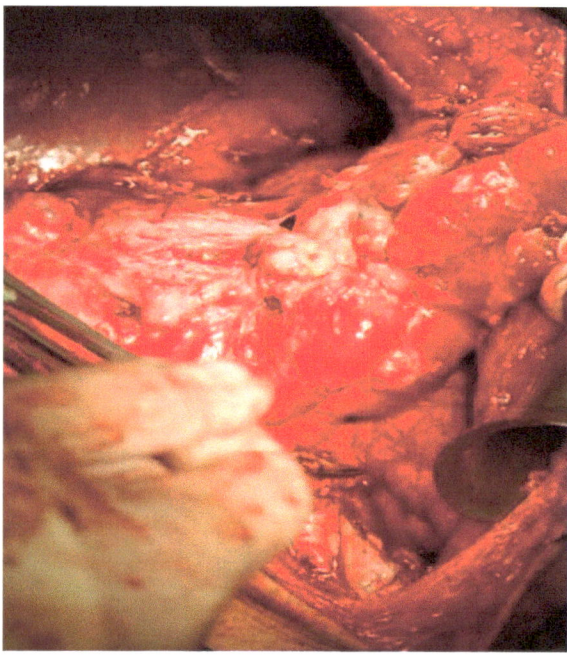

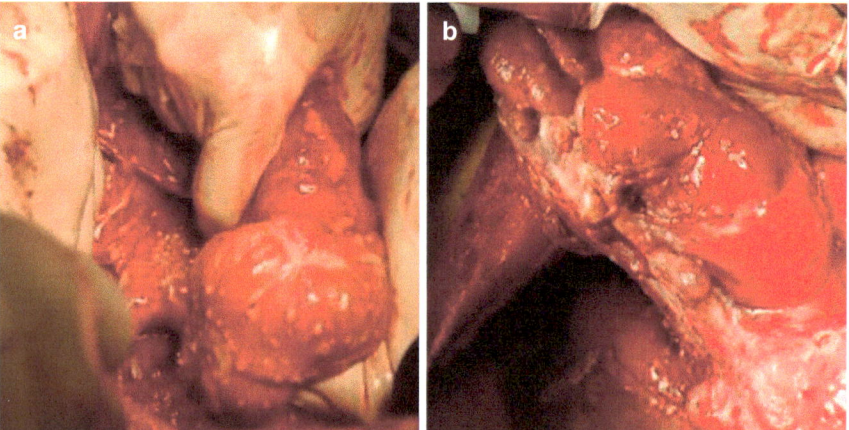

Fig. 1.9 (**a**) Small bowel surfaces are infiltrated with metastatic nodules. (**b**) Small bowel surfaces are infiltrated with metastatic nodules

cytoreduction. Small bowel mesenteric nodules are removed. He had a CC-3 resection and HIPEC. His postoperative period was uneventful. He was discharged on postoperative day 12. He had only 3 months free from symptoms. Then, best palliative care was initiated and he died in the end of April 2016, 22 months after his first diagnosis.

1.4   Discussion

Diagnosis and management of developed small bowel adenocarcinoma (SBA) and even peritoneal metastases (PM) from SBA-associated Crohn's disease (CD) are challenging. Diagnosis of SBA represents difficulties even at early stages due to the lack of specific tumor markers and vague symptoms and limitations of imaging techniques.

So far, there is no any report presenting the PM from SBA-associated CD.

PM of SBA has been reported previously from other groups. These studies are listed in Table 1.2.

Systemic chemotherapy contributes to prolonged survival. A platinum compound has been found to prolong survival than those who received only fluorouracil [20]. One largest study regarding the effects of systemic chemotherapy showed that 30% response rates were detected in metastatic or locally advanced unresectable SBA with a median survival of 11 months [21].

Cytoreductive surgery and hyperthermic intraoperative intraperitoneal chemotherapy gradually gained an acceptance in the management of peritoneal metastasis from other origins. Even though the results are promising, the role of CRS and HIPEC in patients with PM of SBA still remains unclear. Evaluation of these data for efficacy of CRS and HIPEC is challenging because there are still no comparative studies.

The results of CRS and HIPEC in patients with PM of SBA associated with CD are even undefined.

Our patient might have longer survival if the patient underwent CRS and HIPEC or even treated with adjuvant normothermic intraperitoneal chemotherapy during his earlier interventions. These are all remains to be investigated.

Short life expectancy in these patients with present approaches indicates the careful evaluation and to perform new interventions to prolong survival and even cure in patients with PM of SBA associated with CD.

Future studies should clarify the exact role of CRS and HIPEC and intraperitoneal chemotherapy applications in the management of PM from SBA associated with CD.

Table 1.2 Cytoreductive surgery and hyperthermic intraoperative intraperitoneal chemotherapy for PM of patients with small bowel malignancies

Studies performed cytoreductive surgery and HIEPC for peritoneal metastasis of small bowel malignancies				
Authors	Pts number	CRS and HIPEC	Median survival	Overall survival
Sun Y (2013) [14]	17	+	37 months	18.4 months
Jacks SP (2005) [15]				
Marchetini and Sugarbaker (2002) [16]	6	+	12 months	–
Chua TC (2009) [17]	5	+	12 months	–
Elias D(2010) [18]	31	+	47 months	33.8% for 5 years
Liu Y (2016) [19]	21	+	36 months	12% for 5 years

References

1. Ginzburg L, Schneider KM, Dreizin DH, Levinson U. Carcinoma of the jejunum occurring in a case of regional enteritis. Surgery. 1956;39:347–51.
2. Von Roon AC, Reese G, Teare J, Constantinides V, Darzi AW, Tekkis PP. The risk of cancer in patients with Crohn's Disease. Dis Colon Rectum. 2007;50(6):839–55.
3. Dossett LA, White LM, Welch DC, Herline AJ, Muldoon RL, Schwartz DA, Wise PE. Small bowel adenocarcinoma complicating Crohn's disease: case series and review of the literature. Am Surg. 2007;73:1181–7.
4. Widmar M, Greenstein AJ, Sachar DB, Harpaz N, Bauer JJ, Greenstein AJ. Small bowel adenocarcinoma in Crohn's disease. J Gastrointest Surg. 2011;15:797–802.
5. Palascak-Juif V, Bouvier AM, Cosnes J, Flourie B, Bouche O, Cadiot G, Lemann M, Bonaz B, Denet C, Marteau P, Gambiez L, Beaugerie L, Faivre J, Carbonnel F. Small bowel adenocarcinoma in patients with Crohn's disease compared with small bowel adenocarcinoma de novo. Inflamm Bowel Dis. 2005;11(9):828–32.
6. Solem CA, Harmsen WS, Zinsmeister AR, Loftus EV. Small intestinal adenocarcinoma in Crohn's disease: a case-control study. Inflamm Bowel Dis. 2004;10:32–5.
7. Buckley JA, Siegelman SS, Jones B, Fishman EK. The accuracy of CT staging of small bowel adenocarcinoma: CT/pathologic correlation. J Comput Assist Tomogr. 1997;21:986–91.
8. Elsayes KM, Al-Hawary MM, Jagdish J, Ganesh HS, Platt JF. CT enterography: principles, trends, and interpretation of findings. Radiographics. 2010;30(7):1955–70.
9. Engin G. Computed tomography enteroclysis in the diagnosis of intestinal diseases. J Comput Assist Tomogr. 2008;32:9–16.
10. Ikeuchi H, Nakano H, Uchino M, Nakamura M, Matsuoka H, Fukuda Y, Matsumoto T, Takesue Y, Tomita N. Intestinal cancer in Crohn's disease. Hepatogastroenterology. 2008;55(88):2121–4.
11. Shinya T, Inai R, Tanaka T, Akagi N, Sato S, Yoshino T, Kanazawa S. Small bowel neoplasms: enhancement patterns and differentiation using post-contrast multiphasic multidetector CT. Abdom Radiol (NY). 2016; doi:10.1007/soo261-016-0945-y.
12. Watanebe M, Nakano H, Takano E, Miyachi I, Ito M, Kawase K. Gastroenterol Jpn. 1991;26(4):514–22.
13. Greenstein AJ. Cancer in inflammatory bowel disease. Mt Sinai J Med. 2000;67:227–40.
14. Sun Y, Shen P, Stewart JH, Russel GB, Levine EA. Cytoreductive Surgery and hyperthermic intraperitoneal chemotherapy for peritoneal carcinomatosis from small bowel adenocarcinoma. Am Surg. 2013;79:644–8.
15. Jacks SP, Hundley JC, Shen P, Russell GB, Levine EA. Cytoreductive surgery and intraperitoneal hyperthermic chemotherapy for peritoneal carcinomatosis from small bowel adenocarcinoma. J Surg Oncol. 2005;91:112–7.
16. Marchettini P, Sugarbaker PH. Mucinous adenocarcinoma of the small bowel with peritoneal seeding. Eur J Surg Oncol. 2002;28:19–23.
17. Chua TC, Koh JL, Yan TD, Liauw W, Morris DL. Cytoreductive surgery and perioperative intraperitoneal chemotherapy for peritoneal carcinomatosis from small bowel adenocarcinoma. J Surg Oncol. 2005;91:112–7.
18. Elias D, Glehen O, Pocard M, Quenet F, Goere D, Arvieux C, Rat P, Gilly F. Association Francaise de Chirurgie. A comparative study of complete cytoreductive surgery plus intraperitoneal chemotherapy to treat peritoneal dissemination from colon, rectum, small bowel, and nonpseudomyxoma appendix. Ann Surg. 2010;251:896–901.
19. Liu Y, Ishibashi H, Takeshita K, Mizumoto A, Hirano M, Sako S, Takegawa S, Takao N, Ichinose M, Yonemura Y. Cytoreductive surgery and hyperthermic intraperitoneal chemotherapy for peritoneal dissemination from small bowel malignancy: results from a single specialized center. Ann Surg Oncol. 2016 May;23(5):1625–31.

20. Overman MJ, Kopetz S, Wen S, Hoff PM, Fogelman D, Morris J, Abbruzzese JL, Ajani JA, Wolff RA. Chemotherapy with 5-fluorouracil and a platinum compound improves outcomes in metastatic small bowel adenocarcinoma. Cancer. 2008;113(8):2038–45.
21. Fishman PN, Pond GR, Moore MJ, Oza A, Burkes RL, Siu LL, Feld R, Gallinger S, Greig P, Knox JJ. Natural history and chemotherapy effectiveness for advanced adenocarcinoma of the small bowel: a retrospective review of 113 cases. Am J Clin Oncol. 2006;29:225–31.

Chapter 2
Selection of Chemotherapy in Hyperthermic Intraperitoneal Chemotherapy

H.J. Braam and F.J.H. Hoogwater

2.1 Introduction

The peritoneum consists of a layer of mesothelial cells covering all abdominal organs and the abdominopelvic wall. Peritoneal metastases are formed after exfoliation of free tumor cells from a primary tumor invading the peritoneum. Consequently, most peritoneal metastases originate from abdominal organs such as the colon, rectum, stomach, or ovaria. Cancer cells spread in the abdominal cavity resulting from the natural flow of intraperitoneal fluids and subsequently outgrow into multiple nodular metastases on the peritoneum. Peritoneal metastases remain one of the most oncological challenges in current treatment of various intra-abdominal malignancies [1]. Current systemic palliative chemotherapeutic regimes appear to have only a limited effect in treating peritoneal metastases, both in improving survival and decreasing symptoms of peritoneal metastases such as bowel obstruction or the formation of disabling amounts of ascites. New treatment strategies involving cytoreductive surgery combined with hyperthermic intraperitoneal chemotherapy have shown favorable results in numerous intraperitoneal metastasizing intra-abdominal malignancies, such as appendiceal and colorectal cancer. Following the randomized controlled trial by Verwaal et al. [2], cytoreductive surgery combined with hyperthermic intraperitoneal chemotherapy (HIPEC) in patients with limited peritoneal metastases of colorectal cancer (CRC) is now regarded as standard treatment in selected patients (no extraperitoneal disease and sufficient performance status). The goal of cytoreductive surgery (CRS) is to remove all macroscopic malignant disease by performing several visceral resections and peritonectomy procedures.

H.J. Braam (✉) • F.J.H. Hoogwater
Department of Surgery, St. Antonius Hospital, Nieuwegein, The Netherlands

Peritoneal Dissemination Treatment, Istanbul, Istanbul, Turkey
e-mail: h.braam@antoniusziekenhuis.nl

This is followed by a 30–90 min intraperitoneal perfusion of the abdominal cavity using heated chemotherapy. The aim of this so-called hyperthermic intraperitoneal chemotherapy (HIPEC) is to eradicate any remaining microscopic tumor cells. The chemotherapy is generally heated up to 41–43 °C. This is performed for several reasons; first in vitro cancer cells sensitivity is increased in many chemotherapeutic drugs. Additionally, some studies have shown improved pharmacokinetics of chemotherapy in hyperthermic conditions. Currently, various chemotherapeutic drugs, such as mitomycin or cisplatin, are used for HIPEC. Several factors influence the selection of the appropriate drug selection for the use in intraperitoneal chemotherapy. Important drug characteristics are systemic activity in the treating malignancy, concentration-related cytotoxicity, hyperthermic synergy, favorable intraperitoneal pharmacokinetics, adequate tissue penetration, acceptable local and systemic toxicity, and the safety of administration for hospital personnel. Drugs with a direct cytotoxic effect, i.e., not cell cycle specific, will have more potential as in HIPEC the exposure time of the chemotherapeutic drug is limited, and multiple administrations are not feasible in HIPEC. Different chemotherapeutic drugs, and combinations of these, are used for the use in intraperitoneal chemotherapeutic treatment. Table 2.1 gives an overview of current or investigated drugs for HIPEC treatment. The goal of the current chapter is to provide a comprehensive overview on the selection of chemotherapeutic drugs for intraperitoneal chemotherapy in various malignancies.

Table 2.1 Chemotherapy agents and their doses for hyperthermic intraoperative intraperitoneal chemotherapy in peritoneal metastases originated from different origins

Drug	Category	Systemic use	Area under the curve	Dose (mg/m^2)
Carboplatin	Platinum analog	Ovarian, bladder, esophageal, sarcoma	10	300
Cisplatin	Platinum analog	Ovarian, bladder, endometrial esophageal, gastric	6.6 [3]	90
Oxaliplatin	Platinum analog	CRC, ovarian, esophageal, stomach, pancreas	13.2 [3]	460
Doxorubicin	Topoisomerase II inhibitor	Bladder, endometrial sarcoma	78 [4]	15
Mitomycin C	Antibiotic	Stomach, pancreas	24–80 [5–7]	15
Melphalan	Alkylating agent	Ovarian	33 [8]	70
Etoposide	Topoisomerase II inhibitor	Ovarian	47 [9]	25–350
Irinotecan	Topoisomerase I inhibitor	CRC, esophageal, sarcoma, gastric, pancreas	3.7–14.8 [10, 11]	200
Paclitaxel	Taxane derivative	Ovarian, bladder, esophageal, gastric, sarcoma	153–976 [12–15]	
Docetaxel	Taxane derivative	Gastric, bladder esophageal, sarcoma, ovarian	207–387 [16, 17]	45
5-Fluorouracil	Pyrimidine analog	CRC, gastric, pancreas, bladder, esophageal	403–1,400 [6, 7]	650

2.2 Pharmacology

The use of intraperitoneal chemotherapy is more invasive and challenging than conventional intravenous administration. Therefore intraperitoneal administration should have a pharmacologic advantage resulting in an increased cytotoxic effect on peritoneal tumor cells. The rationale of administrating chemotherapeutic drugs through the intraperitoneal route is based on the blood peritoneal barrier. The blood peritoneal barrier results in a decreased uptake of chemotherapy from the intraperitoneal cavity, which permits high concentrations of intraperitoneal chemotherapy with a limited systemic uptake. Consequently, intraperitoneal administration of chemotherapy can result in significant intraperitoneal cytotoxicity with limited systemic side effects. Importantly, selected drugs should have an increased cytotoxicity following dose intensification, resulting in an increased cytotoxicity after intraperitoneal administration.

The blood peritoneal barrier may decrease the effect of intravenous chemotherapy, which may partly explain the limited effect of systemic chemotherapy on peritoneal metastases. Numerous studies have shown the limited effect of systemic chemotherapy on peritoneal metastases. Franko et al. showed in a pooled analysis of two large randomized controlled trials of 2,095 patients with metastasized colorectal cancer treated with modern systemic chemotherapy that patients with peritoneal metastases have a significantly shorter overall and progression-free survival compared to patients with peritoneal metastasis [18]. Population-based data has shown that although there is an increased usage of systemic chemotherapy in patients with peritoneal metastases of colorectal and gastric cancer, the overall survival in the entire patient group has hardly increased, which supports the paradigm that systemic chemotherapy has only a limited effect on peritoneal metastases [19, 20].

The pharmacologic advantage of intraperitoneal administration of chemotherapy can be described by the area under the curve (AUC) ratio. The AUC is defined as the plot of concentration of drug in blood plasma or peritoneal perfusate against time. The AUC ratio is calculated by dividing the AUC in the perfusate by the blood plasma. Thus the AUC ratio reflects the increased exposure of the peritoneum compared to blood plasma, i.e., a high AUC reflects high peritoneal concentrations and presumable high local efficacy. However, one important consideration is that AUC ratio does not reflect tissue penetration. A very high AUC ratio may reflect insufficient tissue penetration resulting in a decreased efficacy. It is difficult to adequately determine the tissue penetration of HIPEC treatment. Some studies have shown a penetration of several millimeters; however, penetration to only a few cell layers has also been described [21, 22]. Furthermore, tissue samples after cessation of the HIPEC are not available. Probably, part of chemotherapy remains incorporated in the tissues surrounding the peritoneal cavity. Rapid systemic metabolism and excretion also influences the AUC ratio. Rapidly metabolized and excreted of the chemotherapeutic drug in the plasma results in less systemic toxicity.

Interestingly, in a study of 145 patients with colorectal or appendiceal carcinomatosis who underwent cytoreductive surgery combined with HIPEC using mitomycin, the number of peritonectomies did not influence the uptake of intraperitoneal chemotherapy [5]. Only large visceral resections such as total colectomies and gastrectomies resulted in a decrease of uptake of intraperitoneal chemotherapy.

As in systemic chemotherapy, dosage of intraperitoneal chemotherapy is currently based on the body surface area of a patient (m^2). As shown by cadaver studies, there is a correlation between the peritoneal surface area and body surface area, and the peritoneal surface area can be estimated by formulas used to calculate body surface area [23]. However, peritoneal surface disease such as pseudomyxoma peritonei may significantly influence the peritoneal surface area; by forming large amounts of mucus, the size of peritoneal area may be increased. Furthermore, dosage on body surface area does not incorporate the volume of the peritoneal cavity, which can also significantly differ inter-individually. The chance of an inadequate dosing in a patient is probably larger when using a fixed dose of chemotherapy per patient (mg). For instance, in a patient with a limited peritoneal surface area, but with a relatively large peritoneal cavity, using a fixed concentration could result in a concentration on the peritoneal surface which is inadequate to induce cytotoxicity. Previous studies have used a standard concentration dosage (mg/l) in HIPEC; this could lead to toxic plasma levels in patients with a relatively large peritoneal surface area. Therefore a concentration based on the body surface of a patient currently seems to be the most appropriate dosing system in HIPEC treatment.

2.3   Colorectal Cancer

In colorectal cancer, mitomycin is the most frequently used and studied drug in the treatment of peritoneal metastases with HIPEC. A first randomized clinical trial to compare CRS with HIPEC using mitomycin vs. systemic chemotherapy showed a survival benefit of 9 months with CRS and HIPEC arm (21.6 versus 12.6 months, $p = 0.032$) [24]. Mitomycin is frequently dosed at 35 mg/m^2 for 90 min HIPEC. Following the fast breakdown of mitomycin, administration is administrated at multiple times during the 90 min HIPEC. At initial stage of HIPEC, half of the dose is administered, and after 30 and 60 min another one-quarter is added to the perfusate. Mitomycin has favorable pharmacokinetics for intraperitoneal usage. Van der Speeten et al. investigated the pharmacokinetics of mitomycin in 145 patients treated with a 90 min HIPEC with a single dose of 15 mg/m^2 [5]. The authors calculated a AUC ratio in these patients of 27. At the start of the perfusion, the peak intraperitoneal concentration was 10 µg/mL, which was significantly higher compared to a peak plasma concentration of 0.25 µg/mL following 30 min of HIPEC. After 90 min of perfusion, in the remaining perfusion fluid 29% of mitomycin was measured and 9% was excreted in the urine.

Intraoperative administration of mitomycin has been shown to be safe and not produce a hazard to the surgical personnel [25]. Consequently, from its cytotoxic effect, local effects such as decreased wound healing and possibly increased rate of postoperative complications, such as anastomotic leakage, are shown in animal studies [26, 27]. However, mitomycin is the widely used drug in HIPEC in large groups of patients, therefore the local toxicity and systemic toxicity of mitomycin are described extensively, showing acceptable morbidity and mortality [28, 29]. In clinical studies, systemic and dose-limiting toxicity in mitomycin is neutropenia; however, in daily clinical practice, this is a relatively rare clinically relevant complication.

In vitro, multiple studies have shown that cytotoxicity of mitomycin is increased using hyperthermia [30, 31]. There is limited data on the clinical relevancy of heat augmentation in HIPEC treatment; however, the appliance of hyperthermia in intraoperative intraperitoneal perfusion is not demanding or costly. Furthermore, no negative side effects of hyperthermia are currently reported.

Following the beneficial effect of oxaliplatin in colorectal cancer both as first-line systemic treatment and as an adjuvant chemotherapeutic drug [32, 33], Elias et al. extensively investigated oxaliplatin as an intraperitoneal chemotherapeutic drug for the use in HIPEC treatment [34, 35]. A pioneering dose escalation study showed that during a 30 min HIPEC a dose of 460 mg/m^2 can be administered safely [36]. They performed HIPEC at an intraperitoneal temperature of 42–44 °C. Additionally, plasma levels of intraperitoneal oxaliplatin (460 mg/m^2) remained below historical reports of plasma levels after systemic administration of oxaliplatin. During intraperitoneal chemotherapy with oxaliplatin, intravenous 5-fluorouracil (400 mg/m^2) and leucovorin (20 mg/m^2) was administered at the start of HIPEC perfusion. This strategy was chosen as oxaliplatin as monotherapy is considered to be relatively ineffective in systemic chemotherapeutic treatment regimens [37].

In early studies, oxaliplatin is used with a 5% dextrose carrier solution, as oxaliplatin is considered to be relatively unstable in chloride-containing solutions. However, recent in vitro studies have shown that degradation of oxaliplatin is limited, less than 10% after 30 min and less than 20% after 2 h [38]. Furthermore, using dextrose as carrier solution has been associated with severe hyperglycemia and electrolyte disturbances [39].

Two studies have compared HIPEC treatment with mitomycin or oxaliplatin. Hompes et al. performed a comparison of 39 patients treated with oxaliplatin and 56 patients with mitomycin [40]. The extent of peritoneal spread was significantly higher in patients treated with oxaliplatin. Neutropenia only occurred in patients treated with mitomycin (26.8%). After statistical correction for the extent of PC, a comparable intra-abdominal complication rate was seen in both groups. In the oxaliplatin group, median recurrence-free survival was 12.2 months and 13.8 months in the mitomycin group ($p = 0.87$). Median overall survival is 37.1 months in the oxaliplatin group and 26.5 months in the mitomycin group ($p = 0.45$). The authors concluded that no clear benefit of either drug could be demonstrated in the study regarding recurrence-free and overall survival.

In a comparison performed by the American Society of Peritoneal Surface Malignancies of 539 patients treated with either mitomycin of oxaliplatin after complete macroscopic cytoreduction, median overall survival was 31.4 months for the oxaliplatin group and 32.7 months for the mitomycin group ($p = 0.925$) [41]. Also a stratified analysis was performed using the peritoneal surface disease severity score (PSDSS), a score incorporating clinical symptoms, extent of peritoneal spread, and histology. In patients with PSDSS 1/2 median overall survival rates was 54.3 months in those receiving mitomycin versus 28.2 months in those receiving oxaliplatin ($p = 0.012$). Median overall survival in PSDSS 3/4 patients was 19.4 months in the mitomycin group versus 30.4 months in oxaliplatin group ($p = 0.427$). The authors conclude that in patients with a low disease burden of colorectal peritoneal metastases mitomycin seems a superior drug compared to oxaliplatin.

2.4   Ovarian Cancer

Primary or interval cytoreductive surgery combined with systemic chemotherapy is regarded as standard treatment in patients with advanced-stage epithelial ovarian cancer. As epithelial ovarian cancer confines to the abdominal cavity for much of its natural history, administering chemotherapy directly into the peritoneal cavity is attractive. In ovarian cancer, many studies have focused on multiple administrations through catheters of intraperitoneal chemotherapy following cytoreductive surgery. Meta-analysis of nine randomized controlled trials, investigating the beneficial effect of adding intraperitoneal chemotherapy to a standard treatment regime, has shown that intraperitoneal chemotherapy increases progression-free and overall survival in advanced ovarian cancer [42]. However, catheter-related adverse events are prevalent, and major complications have been described [43, 44]. Adverse events result in discontinuation of therapy in more than half of patients, before completing six cycles of intraperitoneal chemotherapy [45]. Hyperthermic intraoperative intraperitoneal chemotherapy may overcome the problems associated with repetitive catheter-based intraperitoneal chemotherapy. A meta-analysis of 37 studies investigating cytoreductive surgery and HIPEC in advanced and recurrent epithelial ovarian cancer showed improved survival rates both compared to CRS alone. Furthermore in this analysis, morbidity and mortality rates were similar [46].

Different chemotherapeutic drugs are used from HIPEC treatment in ovarian cancer. Cisplatin is currently the most frequent drug for intraperitoneal use in ovarian cancer (REFS). Selection of systemic chemotherapy in ovarian cancer is based on the platinum resistance or sensitivity [47]. In a randomized controlled trial by Spiliotis et al., cisplatin and paclitaxel were used in platinum-sensitive disease and doxorubicin and paclitaxel or mitomycin in platinum-resistant disease [48]. Survival was significantly better in the HIPEC group with 26.7 months compared to 13.4 months in the group only undergoing cytoreductive surgery ($p < 0.006$). In the group treated with HIPEC, survival was not different between patients with platinum-sensitive disease or platinum-resistant disease (26.6 vs. 26.8 months). An analysis of the HYPER-O registry, an internet-based registry collecting data from collaborating institutions, compared the effect of different chemotherapy agents on survival [49]. In the entire group of patients, carboplatin was associated with an improved overall survival compared to mitomycin ($p = 0.003$) or cisplatin ($p = 0.003$). When comparing patients with platinum-sensitive recurrent ovarian cancer, carboplatin resulted in a significantly improved survival versus cisplatin ($p = 0.012$) and mitomycin ($p = 0.011$). There was no significant difference between chemotherapeutic drugs in platinum-resistant disease. This study shows that platinum resistance may also be of importance in ovarian cancer treatment with HIPEC. Bakrin et al. described 246 prospectively studied patients with ovarian cancer undergoing HIPEC with cisplatin in 95.5% of procedures, alone or in combination with doxorubicin or mitomycin. Median overall survival was 48 months for patients with platinum-resistant recurrent disease and 52 months for patients with platinum-sensitive recurrent disease, which is superior to historically reported survival rates in this patient group [50]. Currently five randomized controlled trials are being performed investigating the role of HIPEC in ovarian cancer; all are using cisplatin 75–100 mg/m^2, and one added paclitaxel 175 mg/m^2 to their intraperitoneal drug regime [51].

2.5 Gastric Cancer

In gastric cancer after potentially curative treatment, locoregional and peritoneal recurrences are the most frequent sites of treatment failure [52]. In patients with peritoneal carcinomatosis of gastric cancer, survival is poor, with a median survival of about 3 months [53]. In gastric cancer, many randomized controlled trials have been performed in Asia investigating the role of prophylactic HIPEC in patients at high risk for intraperitoneal recurrence. A recent meta-analysis concluded that this treatment may prevent local recurrence and improve survival [54]. In patients with established peritoneal metastases, one randomized controlled trial has been performed investigating the efficacy and safety of HIPEC with cisplatin and mitomycin. This study showed a significant median overall survival improvement in cytoreductive surgery combined with HIPEC group compared to cytoreductive surgery alone (11.0 versus 6.5 months, $p = 0.046$) [55]. Complication rates did not differ in both groups.

Originating from its widespread usage and experience in other malignancies, mitomycin C is the most frequently investigated drug in HIPEC for gastric cancer. Mitomycin C has only limited effect in systemic treatment of gastric cancer, therefore other agents should be investigated for the use in HIPEC in gastric cancer patients.

The platinum-based agents oxaliplatin and cisplatin have both been investigated for HIPEC in gastric cancer. In vitro and in systemic treatment, oxaliplatin seems a more potent drug in gastric cancer [56, 57]. Furthermore, pharmacological advantages after intraperitoneal administration have been described for oxaliplatin compared to cisplatin [3, 58]. The adverse effects of cisplatin and oxaliplatin following intraperitoneal administration are acceptable, and limited hematological toxicity has been described [59, 60]. There are currently no studies in humans comparing intraperitoneal cisplatin and oxaliplatin. An enhanced in vitro efficacy in hyperthermic conditions has been demonstrated for oxaliplatin and cisplatin.

Systemic administration of taxane alkaloids has shown improved response rates in the systemic treatment of gastric cancer [61, 62]. The taxane alkaloids docetaxel and paclitaxel are dissolved in micellar preparations polysorbate 80 and Cremophor EL as these agents are barely soluble in other solvents. Preclinical data shows that the cell permeability of paclitaxel is significantly inhibited by its solvent, resulting in decreased tumor and cell uptake. Therefore docetaxel seems a more appropriate candidate for intraperitoneal perfusion [63]. Several studies have shown the favorable pharmacokinetics of intraperitoneally administered taxanes with high AUC ratios but with adequate tissue penetration [12, 13, 15, 64]. Additionally, several studies have shown the safety of using taxanes for HIPEC treatment [17, 65].

2.6   Future Perspectives

The many variables in HIPEC such as dosage, extent of cytoreduction, timing of HIPEC, temperature, duration of perfusion, carrier solution, and pharmacokinetics warrant more experimental and clinical studies to investigate the role of each individual parameters and select the most suitable HIPEC regime for each different type of malignancy. Ideally, individual analysis on tumor biology and underlying molecular mechanisms could result in the development of a patient-tailored HIPEC schedule. For instance, de Cuba et al. have described that high VEGF expression levels in peritoneal metastases of CRC results in a worse overall survival after cytoreductive surgery and HIPEC [66]. The authors suggest that VEGF expression could help identify patients at risk for early recurrence. VEGF expression could be a useful parameter in selecting CRC patients for HIPEC treatment. Additionally, in patients with high VEGF expression, enhanced surveillance programs could be initiated to detect and treat early recurrence. In a study by the same group, apart from simplified peritoneal cancer index and age, VEGF expression levels and epithelial VCAN expression levels were independently associated with overall survival following HIPEC [67]. Furthermore, these biomarkers may be a potential target for adjuvant treatment strategies. To improve the outcome in treatment of peritoneal metastases, additional studies on the selection of the appropriate chemotherapeutic drug is of importance.

References

1. Lambert LA. Looking up: recent advances in understanding and treating peritoneal carcinomatosis. CA Cancer J Clin. 2015;65:284–98.
2. Verwaal VJ, Bruin S, Boot H, van Slooten G, van Tinteren H. 8-year follow-up of randomized trial: cytoreduction and hyperthermic intraperitoneal chemotherapy versus systemic chemotherapy in patients with peritoneal carcinomatosis of colorectal cancer. Ann Surg Oncol. 2008;15:2426–32.

3. Braam HJ, Schellens JH, Boot H, van Sandick JW, Knibbe CA, Boerma D, van Ramshorst B. Selection of chemotherapy for hyperthermic intraperitoneal use in gastric cancer. Crit Rev Oncol Hematol. 2015;95:282–96.
4. Sugarbaker PH, Van der Speeten K, Anthony Stuart O, Chang D. Impact of surgical and clinical factors on the pharmacology of intraperitoneal doxorubicin in 145 patients with peritoneal carcinomatosis. Eur J Surg Oncol. 2011;37:719–26.
5. Van der Speeten K, Stuart OA, Chang D, Mahteme H, Sugarbaker PH. Changes induced by surgical and clinical factors in the pharmacology of intraperitoneal mitomycin C in 145 patients with peritoneal carcinomatosis. Cancer Chemother Pharmacol. 2011;68:147–56.
6. Kuzuya T, Yamauchi M, Ito A, Hasegawa M, Hasegawa T, Nabeshima T. Pharmacokinetic characteristics of 5-fluorouracil and mitomycin C in intraperitoneal chemotherapy. J Pharm Pharmacol. 1994;46:685–9.
7. Jacquet P, Averbach A, Stuart OA, Chang D, Sugarbaker PH. Hyperthermic intraperitoneal doxorubicin: pharmacokinetics, metabolism, and tissue distribution in a rat model. Cancer Chemother Pharmacol. 1998;41:147–54.
8. Sugarbaker PH, Stuart OA. Pharmacokinetic and phase II study of heated intraoperative intraperitoneal melphalan. Cancer Chemother Pharmacol. 2007;59:151–5.
9. O'Dwyer PJ, LaCreta FP, Daugherty JP, Hogan M, Rosenblum NG, O'Dwyer JL, Comis RL. Phase I pharmacokinetic study of intraperitoneal etoposide. Cancer Res. 1991;51:2041–6.
10. Guichard S, Chatelut E, Lochon I, Bugat R, Mahjoubi M, Canal P. Comparison of the pharmacokinetics and efficacy of irinotecan after administration by the intravenous versus intraperitoneal route in mice. Cancer Chemother Pharmacol. 1998;42:165–70.
11. Turcotte S, Sideris L, Younan R, Drolet P, Dube P. Pharmacokinetics of intraperitoneal irinotecan in a pig model. J Surg Oncol. 2010;101:637–42.
12. Kamijo Y, Ito C, Nomura M, Sai Y, Miyamoto K. Surfactants influence the distribution of taxanes in peritoneal dissemination tumor-bearing rats. Cancer Lett. 2010;287:182–6.
13. Shimada T, Nomura M, Yokogawa K, Endo Y, Sasaki T, Miyamoto K, Yonemura Y. Pharmacokinetic advantage of intraperitoneal injection of docetaxel in the treatment for peritoneal dissemination of cancer in mice. J Pharm Pharmacol. 2005;57:177–81.
14. Yonemura Y, Endou Y, Bando E, et al. Effect of intraperitoneal administration of docetaxel on peritoneal dissemination of gastric cancer. Cancer Lett. 2004;210:189–96.
15. Marchettini P, Stuart OA, Mohamed F, Yoo D, Sugarbaker PH. Docetaxel: pharmacokinetics and tissue levels after intraperitoneal and intravenous administration in a rat model. Cancer Chemother Pharmacol. 2002;49:499–503.
16. de Bree E, Rosing H, Beijnen JH, Romanos J, Michalakis J, Georgoulias V, Tsiftsis DD. Pharmacokinetic study of docetaxel in intraoperative hyperthermic i.p. chemotherapy for ovarian cancer. Anti-Cancer Drugs. 2003;14:103–10.
17. de Bree E, Rosing H, Filis D, et al. Cytoreductive surgery and intraoperative hyperthermic intraperitoneal chemotherapy with paclitaxel: a clinical and pharmacokinetic study. Ann Surg Oncol. 2008;15:1183–92.
18. Franko J, Shi Q, Goldman CD, et al. Treatment of colorectal peritoneal carcinomatosis with systemic chemotherapy: a pooled analysis of north central cancer treatment group phase III trials N9741 and N9841. J Clin Oncol. 2012;30:263–7.
19. Klaver YL, Lemmens VE, Creemers GJ, Rutten HJ, Nienhuijs SW, de Hingh IH. Population-based survival of patients with peritoneal carcinomatosis from colorectal origin in the era of increasing use of palliative chemotherapy. Ann Oncol. 2011;22:2250–6.
20. Bernards N, Creemers GJ, Nieuwenhuijzen GA, Bosscha K, Pruijt JF, Lemmens VE. No improvement in median survival for patients with metastatic gastric cancer despite increased use of chemotherapy. Ann Oncol. 2013;24:3056–60.
21. Ansaloni L, Coccolini F, Morosi L, et al. Pharmacokinetics of concomitant cisplatin and paclitaxel administered by hyperthermic intraperitoneal chemotherapy to patients with peritoneal carcinomatosis from epithelial ovarian cancer. Br J Cancer. 2015;112:306–12.
22. Los G, Mutsaers PH, van der Vijgh WJ, Baldew GS, de Graaf PW, McVie JG. Direct diffusion of cis-diamminedichloroplatinum(II) in intraperitoneal rat tumors after intraperitoneal chemotherapy: a comparison with systemic chemotherapy. Cancer Res. 1989;49:3380–4.

23. Albanese AM, Albanese EF, Mino JH, Gomez E, Gomez M, Zandomeni M, Merlo AB. Peritoneal surface area: measurements of 40 structures covered by peritoneum: correlation between total peritoneal surface area and the surface calculated by formulas. Surg Radiol Anat. 2009;31:369–77.
24. Verwaal VJ, van Ruth S, de Bree E, van Sloothen GW, van Tinteren H, Boot H, Zoetmulder FA. Randomized trial of cytoreduction and hyperthermic intraperitoneal chemotherapy versus systemic chemotherapy and palliative surgery in patients with peritoneal carcinomatosis of colorectal cancer. J Clin Oncol. 2003;21:3737–43.
25. Schmid K, Boettcher MI, Pelz JO, Meyer T, Korinth G, Angerer J, Drexler H. Investigations on safety of hyperthermic intraoperative intraperitoneal chemotherapy (HIPEC) with Mitomycin C. Eur J Surg Oncol. 2006;32:1222–5.
26. Aarts F, Bleichrodt RP, de Man B, Lomme R, Boerman OC, Hendriks T. The effects of adjuvant experimental radioimmunotherapy and hyperthermic intraperitoneal chemotherapy on intestinal and abdominal healing after cytoreductive surgery for peritoneal carcinomatosis in the rat. Ann Surg Oncol. 2008;15:3299–307.
27. Pelz JO, Doerfer J, Decker M, Dimmler A, Hohenberger W, Meyer T. Hyperthermic intraperitoneal chemoperfusion (HIPEC) decrease wound strength of colonic anastomosis in a rat model. Int J Color Dis. 2007;22:941–7.
28. Baratti D, Kusamura S, Pietrantonio F, Guaglio M, Niger M, Deraco M. Progress in treatments for colorectal cancer peritoneal metastases during the years 2010–2015. A systematic review. Crit Rev Oncol Hematol. 2016;100:209–22.
29. Chua TC, Yan TD, Saxena A, Morris DL. Should the treatment of peritoneal carcinomatosis by cytoreductive surgery and hyperthermic intraperitoneal chemotherapy still be regarded as a highly morbid procedure?: a systematic review of morbidity and mortality. Ann Surg. 2009;249:900–7.
30. Murakami A, Koga S, Maeta M. Thermochemosensitivity: augmentation by hyperthermia of cytotoxicity of anticancer drugs against human colorectal cancers, measured by the human tumor clonogenic assay. Oncology. 1988;45:236–41.
31. Watanabe M, Tanaka R, Hondo H, Kuroki M. Effects of antineoplastic agents and hyperthermia on cytotoxicity toward chronically hypoxic glioma cells. Int J Hyperth. 1992;8:131–8.
32. Andre T, Boni C, Mounedji-Boudiaf L, et al. Oxaliplatin, fluorouracil, and leucovorin as adjuvant treatment for colon cancer. N Engl J Med. 2004;350:2343–51.
33. de Gramont A, Figer A, Seymour M, et al. Leucovorin and fluorouracil with or without oxaliplatin as first-line treatment in advanced colorectal cancer. J Clin Oncol. 2000;18:2938–47.
34. Elias D, Goere D, Blot F, Billard V, Pocard M, Kohneh-Shahri N, Raynard B. Optimization of hyperthermic intraperitoneal chemotherapy with oxaliplatin plus irinotecan at 43 degrees C after compete cytoreductive surgery: mortality and morbidity in 106 consecutive patients. Ann Surg Oncol. 2007;14:1818–24.
35. Elias D, El Otmany A, Bonnay M, et al. Human pharmacokinetic study of heated intraperitoneal oxaliplatin in increasingly hypotonic solutions after complete resection of peritoneal carcinomatosis. Oncology. 2002;63:346–52.
36. Elias D, Bonnay M, Puizillou JM, et al. Heated intra-operative intraperitoneal oxaliplatin after complete resection of peritoneal carcinomatosis: pharmacokinetics and tissue distribution. Ann Oncol. 2002;13:267–72.
37. Rothenberg ML, Oza AM, Bigelow RH, et al. Superiority of oxaliplatin and fluorouracil-leucovorin compared with either therapy alone in patients with progressive colorectal cancer after irinotecan and fluorouracil-leucovorin: interim results of a phase III trial. J Clin Oncol. 2003;21:2059–69.
38. Mehta AM, Van den Hoven JM, Rosing H, et al. Stability of oxaliplatin in chloride-containing carrier solutions used in hyperthermic intraperitoneal chemotherapy. Int J Pharm. 2015;479:23–7.
39. De Somer F, Ceelen W, Delanghe J, De Smet D, Vanackere M, Pattyn P, Mortier E. Severe hyponatremia, hyperglycemia, and hyperlactatemia are associated with intraoperative hyperthermic intraperitoneal chemoperfusion with oxaliplatin. Perit Dial Int. 2008;28:61–6.

40. Hompes D, D'Hoore A, Wolthuis A, Fieuws S, Mirck B, Bruin S, Verwaal V. The use of Oxaliplatin or Mitomycin C in HIPEC treatment for peritoneal carcinomatosis from colorectal cancer: a comparative study. J Surg Oncol. 2014;109:527–32.
41. Prada-Villaverde A, Esquivel J, Lowy AM, et al. The American Society of Peritoneal Surface Malignancies evaluation of HIPEC with Mitomycin C versus Oxaliplatin in 539 patients with colon cancer undergoing a complete cytoreductive surgery. J Surg Oncol. 2014;110:779–85.
42. Jaaback K, Johnson N, Lawrie TA. Intraperitoneal chemotherapy for the initial management of primary epithelial ovarian cancer. Cochrane Database Syst Rev. 2016;(1):CD005340. doi:CD005340.
43. Polyzos A, Tsavaris N, Kosmas C, et al. A comparative study of intraperitoneal carboplatin versus intravenous carboplatin with intravenous cyclophosphamide in both arms as initial chemotherapy for stage III ovarian cancer. Oncology. 1999;56:291–6.
44. Yen MS, Juang CM, Lai CR, Chao GC, Ng HT, Yuan CC. Intraperitoneal cisplatin-based chemotherapy vs. intravenous cisplatin-based chemotherapy for stage III optimally cytoreduced epithelial ovarian cancer. Int J Gynaecol Obstet. 2001;72:55–60.
45. Armstrong DK, Bundy B, Wenzel L, et al. Intraperitoneal cisplatin and paclitaxel in ovarian cancer. N Engl J Med. 2006;354:34–43.
46. Huo YR, Richards A, Liauw W, Morris DL. Hyperthermic intraperitoneal chemotherapy (HIPEC) and cytoreductive surgery (CRS) in ovarian cancer: a systematic review and meta-analysis. Eur J Surg Oncol. 2015;41:1578–89.
47. Gore ME, Fryatt I, Wiltshaw E, Dawson T, Robinson BA, Calvert AH. Cisplatin/carboplatin cross-resistance in ovarian cancer. Br J Cancer. 1989;60:767–9.
48. Spiliotis J, Halkia E, Lianos E, Kalantzi N, Grivas A, Efstathiou E, Giassas S. Cytoreductive surgery and HIPEC in recurrent epithelial ovarian cancer: a prospective randomized phase III study. Ann Surg Oncol. 2015;22:1570–5.
49. Helm CW, Richard SD, Pan J, et al. Hyperthermic intraperitoneal chemotherapy in ovarian cancer: first report of the HYPER-O registry. Int J Gynecol Cancer. 2010;20:61–9.
50. Bakrin N, Cotte E, Golfier F, et al. Cytoreductive surgery and hyperthermic intraperitoneal chemotherapy (HIPEC) for persistent and recurrent advanced ovarian carcinoma: a multi-center, prospective study of 246 patients. Ann Surg Oncol. 2012;19:4052–8.
51. van Driel WJ, Lok CA, Verwaal V, Sonke GS. The role of hyperthermic intraperitoneal intraoperative chemotherapy in ovarian cancer. Curr Treat Options in Oncol. 2015;16:14. 015-0329-5
52. Yoo CH, Noh SH, Shin DW, Choi SH, Min JS. Recurrence following curative resection for gastric carcinoma. Br J Surg. 2000;87:236–42.
53. Sadeghi B, Arvieux C, Glehen O, et al. Peritoneal carcinomatosis from non-gynecologic malignancies: results of the EVOCAPE 1 multicentric prospective study. Cancer. 2000;88:358–63.
54. Sun J, Song Y, Wang Z, et al. Benefits of hyperthermic intraperitoneal chemotherapy for patients with serosal invasion in gastric cancer: a meta-analysis of the randomized controlled trials. BMC Cancer. 2012;12:526. 2407-12-526
55. Yang XJ, Huang CQ, Suo T, et al. Cytoreductive surgery and hyperthermic intraperitoneal chemotherapy improves survival of patients with peritoneal carcinomatosis from gastric cancer: final results of a phase III randomized clinical trial. Ann Surg Oncol. 2011;18:1575–81.
56. Montagnani F, Turrisi G, Marinozzi C, Aliberti C, Fiorentini G. Effectiveness and safety of oxaliplatin compared to cisplatin for advanced, unresectable gastric cancer: a systematic review and meta-analysis. Gastric Cancer. 2011;14:50–5.
57. Eriguchi M, Nonaka Y, Yanagie H, Yoshizaki I, Takeda Y, Sekiguchi M. A molecular biological study of anti-tumor mechanisms of an anti-cancer agent Oxaliplatin against established human gastric cancer cell lines. Biochem Pharmacol. 2003;57:412–5.
58. Los G, Mutsaers PH, Ruevekamp M, McVie JG. The use of oxaliplatin versus cisplatin in intraperitoneal chemotherapy in cancers restricted to the peritoneal cavity in the rat. Cancer Lett. 1990;51:109–17.
59. Wu XJ, Yuan P, Li ZY et al. Cytoreductive surgery and hyperthermic intraperitoneal chemotherapy improves the survival of gastric cancer patients with ovarian metastasis and peritoneal dissemination. Tumour Biol. 2013;34(1):463–9.

60. Votanopoulos K, Ihemelandu C, Shen P, Stewart J, Russell G, Levine EA. A comparison of hematologic toxicity profiles after heated intraperitoneal chemotherapy with oxaliplatin and mitomycin C. J Surg Res. 2013;179:e133–9.
61. Chen XL, Chen XZ, Yang C, et al. Docetaxel, cisplatin and fluorouracil (DCF) regimen compared with non-taxane-containing palliative chemotherapy for gastric carcinoma: a systematic review and meta-analysis. PLoS One. 2013;8:e60320.
62. Hironaka S, Zenda S, Boku N, Fukutomi A, Yoshino T, Onozawa Y. Weekly paclitaxel as second-line chemotherapy for advanced or recurrent gastric cancer. Gastric Cancer. 2006;9:14–8.
63. Miyamoto K, Shimada T, Sawamoto K, Sai Y, Yonemura Y. Disposition kinetics of taxanes in peritoneal dissemination. Gastroenterol Res Pract. 2012;2012:963403.
64. Morgan Jr RJ, Doroshow JH, Synold T, et al. Phase I trial of intraperitoneal docetaxel in the treatment of advanced malignancies primarily confined to the peritoneal cavity: dose-limiting toxicity and pharmacokinetics. Clin Cancer Res. 2003;9:5896–901.
65. de Bree E, Romanos J, Michalakis J, Relakis K, Georgoulias V, Melissas J, Tsiftsis DD. Intraoperative hyperthermic intraperitoneal chemotherapy with docetaxel as second-line treatment for peritoneal carcinomatosis of gynaecological origin. Anticancer Res. 2003;23:3019–27.
66. de Cuba EM, de Hingh IH, Sluiter NR, et al. Angiogenesis-related markers and prognosis after cytoreductive surgery and hyperthermic intraperitoneal chemotherapy for metastatic colorectal cancer. Ann Surg Oncol. 2016;23:1601–8.
67. Sluiter NR, de Cuba EM, Kwakman R, et al. Versican and vascular endothelial growth factor expression levels in peritoneal metastases from colorectal cancer are associated with survival after cytoreductive surgery and hyperthermic intraperitoneal chemotherapy. Clin Exp Metastasis. 2016;33:297–307.

Chapter 3
Treatment of Pseudomyxoma Peritonei from Non-appendiceal Primary Sites

Paul H. Sugarbaker

3.1 Introduction

Fann and colleagues reported that pseudomyxoma peritonei is a rare condition with a reported incidence of approximately one patient per million per year [1].

This is a condition characterized by mucinous ascites and tumor that is redistributed throughout the abdomen and pelvis in a characteristic manner. The largest volume of ascites and formed tumor is beneath the diaphragms, within the pelvis, and infiltrating the greater and lesser omentum [2]. The characteristic "omental cake" is not from neoplastic invasion of the omental tissue but results from phagocytic engulfment of mucinous tumor cells by the omental cells. The bowel, especially the small bowel, is relatively spared by formed mucinous tumor but can be adjacent to mucinous ascites. Usually, these mucinous neoplasms are low grade and minimally aggressive; however, moderate-grade adenocarcinoma can result in a similar clinical picture. Cytoreductive surgery using parietal peritonectomy and visceral resection can sometimes result in complete visible resection of the mucinous neoplasm.

In most pseudomyxoma peritonei cases, this condition is associated with an appendiceal mucinous malignancy [3]. However, there may be a wide variety of rare primary sites. The pancreas has been identified as a primary site due to a colloid carcinoma [4]. Also, Zanelli et al. reported a pseudomyxoma peritonei patient after resection of an intraductal papillary mucinous neoplasm of the pancreas [5]. Frantz's tumor of the pancreas has been a cause of pseudomyxoma peritonei [6]. There are also reports of pseudomyxoma peritonei from tumors of urachus [7], small bowel [8], gallbladder and bile ducts [9], fallopian tubes [10], stomach [11], and Hirschsprung's disease [12]. In 1981, an infant who had a mucinous ascites

P.H. Sugarbaker, MD, FACS, FRCS
Center for Gastrointestinal Malignancies, Program in Peritoneal Surface, Oncology,
MedStar Washington Hospital Center, 106 Irving St., NW, Suite 3900,
Washington, DC 20010, USA
e-mail: Paul.Sugarbaker@medstar.net

© Springer International Publishing AG 2017   23
E. Canbay (ed.), *Unusual Cases in Peritoneal Surface Malignancies*,
DOI 10.1007/978-3-319-51523-6_3

associated with an adenomyoma of the pylorus was reported [13]. In these reports, mucus-producing epithelial cells were thought to have been seeded directly into the peritoneal cavity and resulted in pseudomyxoma peritonei. These reports suggest that extreme care to prevent seeding of adenomatous cells into the free peritoneal cavity is warranted. If such spillage does occur, thorough washing of the peritoneal surfaces at risk with a cytocidal agent is necessary [14].

Also, there are reports of extra-abdominal tumors such as adenocarcinoma of the lung or colloid carcinoma of the breast as the primary site of intraperitoneal pseudomyxoma peritonei [15, 16]. Zanarini and Sugarbaker reported on patients with myxoid liposarcoma of the extremity who developed peritoneal myxoid sarcomatosis [17]. Together, these unusual cases show that mucinous tumors from a large number of primary sites can cause pseudomyxoma peritonei. The common features of all these tumors that may cause pseudomyxoma peritonei are a less invasive histopathology and a prominent mucus production. The slow progression of the disease and a mucoid ascites allow the characteristic pattern of peritoneal distribution and are common to all these malignancies. This is because the peristaltic activity of the small intestine limits implantation on the visceral peritoneum.

The goal of this manuscript is to review the world's experience with cytoreductive surgery (CRS) and hyperthermic intraoperative chemotherapy (HIPEC) for patients with unusual abdominal and pelvic neoplasms causing pseudomyxoma peritonei that satisfy the criteria for long-term benefit. This report will be structured as a series of case reports followed by a literature review regarding the particular rare PM tissue type that was treated. From these data, other peritoneal surface oncology centers may wish to offer CRS and HIPEC to patients with similar prognostic features.

3.2 Pseudomyxoma Peritonei from Mucinous Urachal Neoplasms

A common non-appendiceal primary site for pseudomyxoma peritonei is the urachus. This section of the manuscript begins with the presentation of a patient successfully managed by CRS and HIPEC. This is followed by a literature review of the world's experience with this disease treated definitively by CRS and HIPEC.

3.2.1 Case Report

A 47-year-old man was evaluated at our institution after abdominal and pelvic CT suggested a diagnosis of mucinous peritoneal metastases (PM). The patient had intermittently experienced the urination of mucus for 8 years. One year prior to diagnosis, he noted increasing abdominal girth and abdominal cramping. Six months prior to diagnosis of PM, a left inguinal hernia was repaired using a laparoscopic approach with the insertion of mesh.

Computed tomography showed a cystic mass directly above the bladder and mucinous PM with a distribution pattern characteristic of pseudomyxoma peritonei (Figs. 3.1, 3.2, and 3.3). A CT-guided biopsy of the omentum showed mildly atypical epithelial cells. A cystoscopy showed a small defect at the dome of the bladder and copious mucus in the bladder, but no tumor mass was evident. A laparoscopy was performed, which showed mucinous tumor located throughout the abdomen and pelvis and distributed in a characteristic fashion with large-volume disease beneath the right and left hemidiaphragms, omental caking, and an extensive mucoid fluid accumulation within the pelvis. Tumor marker studies showed a cancer antigen 19-9 (CA 19-9) level of 594 U/mL and carcinoembryonic antigen (CEA) level of 14 ng/mL.

The patient was taken to the operating room in February 2006. At the time of surgery, the primary tumor was a supravesical mass that communicated with the bladder through a patent urachus and could be dissected clear of the bladder with a

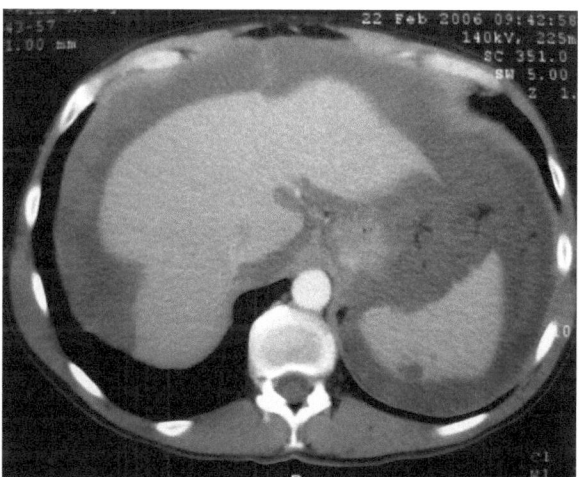

Fig. 3.1 CT scan in a patient with urachal cancer through the upper abdomen showing large volume disease in the right upper quadrant, left upper quadrant, and lesser omentum (From Sugarbaker [59])

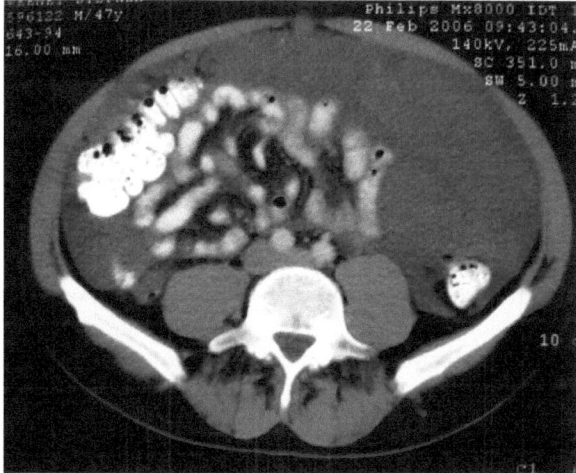

Fig. 3.2 CT scan in a patient with urachal cancer through mid-abdomen showing the "omental cake" characteristic of pseudomyxoma peritonei. The small bowel is compartmentalized beneath the omental cake (From Sugarbaker [59], with permission)

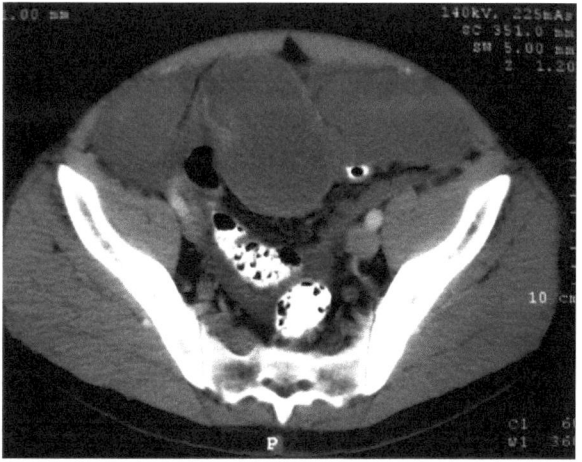

Fig. 3.3 CT scan in a patient with urachal cancer through the lower abdomen showing a cystic mass directly above the bladder (From Sugarbaker [59], with permission)

negative margin. Large volumes of intravesical mucus were suctioned through the opening of the dome of the bladder. No other bladder abnormalities were identified. The appendix, dissected free of the surrounding tissue, was determined to be normal. The findings at surgery showed extensive tumor infiltrating the omentum, beneath hemidiaphragms, and in the pelvis. The small bowel was free of disease (Fig. 3.4).

Cytoreductive surgery required total anterior parietal peritonectomy, right upper quadrant peritonectomy, left upper quadrant peritonectomy, greater and lesser omentectomy, right colectomy, and pelvic peritonectomy including a rectosigmoid colectomy [18, 19]. Segmental cystectomy and closure of the bladder were performed. The tumor, widely distributed within the abdomen and pelvis, was reduced to no visible evidence of disease by CRS. A diverting ileostomy was performed to protect a low colorectal anastomosis. The patient received hyperthermic intraperitoneal mitomycin C (15 mg/m^2) and doxorubicin (15 mg/m^2) and simultaneous bolus intravenous 5-fluorouracil at 600 mg/m^2 and leucovorin at 20 mg/m^2 in the operating room. Tubes and drains were positioned so that patient could receive early postoperative intraperitoneal 5-fluorouracil using 600 mg/m^2 for 4 days.

Histopathologic examination showed a well-differentiated mucinous adenocarcinoma (Fig. 3.5). The patient's postoperative course was uneventful. The ileostomy was closed 1 year later. During this procedure, four small tumor nodules were visualized and removed without difficulty. In 2010, the patient had an abnormal CT 4 years after his definitive procedure. A repeat complete cytoreductive surgery (CCRS) was possible along with additional HIPEC. In 2014, a solitary recurrence in the epigastric region was shown on CT. Radiation therapy was used to control progression. However, in 2015 the mass again began to expand and interfere with gastric function. A left upper quadrant exenterative procedure with total gastrectomy was able to achieve complete resection. Currently, at 10-year post-first procedure, the patient is free of disease.

Fig. 3.4 Intraoperative photograph in a patient with urachal cancer showing the omental cake with normal-appearing small bowel beneath (From Sugarbaker [59], with permission)

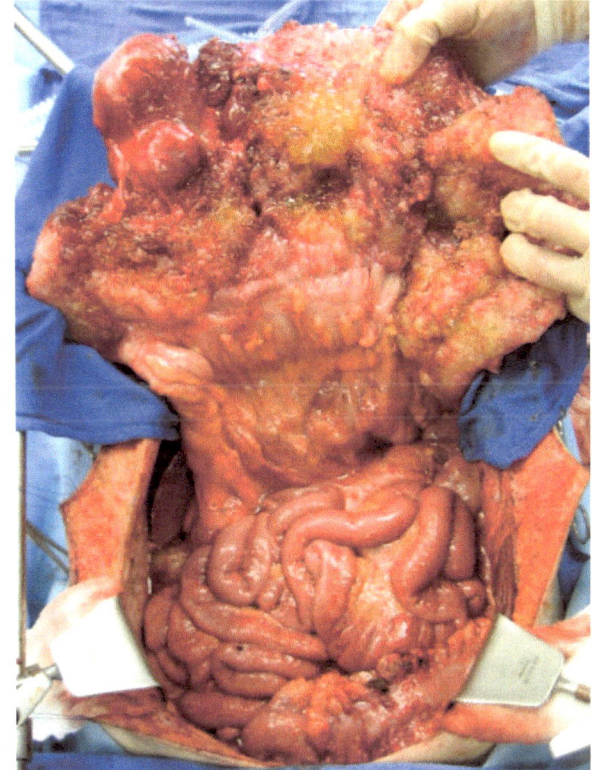

Fig. 3.5 Photomicrograph from a patient with urachal cancer of the wall of the primary tumor mass showed a well-differentiated mucinous malignancy (hematoxylin and eosin ×400) (From Sugarbaker [59])

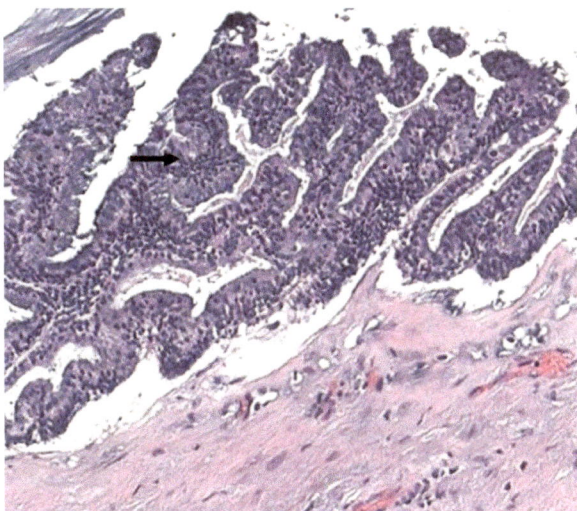

3.2.2   Discussion

The medical literature was searched using PubMed for publications that reported a urachal adenocarcinoma concomitant with PM. The results of this survey are presented in Table 3.1 [7, 12, 19–28]. Mendeloff and McSwain recognized a direct relationship of mucinous PM and the urachal primary cancer [7]. Loggie et al. was the first to report a definitive treatment plan for the local-regional (LR) component of this disease [20]. In that patient, systemic metastases became evident at 20 months after diagnosis; the large-volume intraperitoneal component of the disease never recurred despite systemic progression of disease. Perioperative chemotherapy was used in the report by de Bree as well as in four of our five patients [12, 24]. The patient reported by de Bree et al. was alive and well at 9 years after treatment (personal communication).

3.2.3   Diagnosis of Urachal Pseudomyxoma Peritonei

In the patients reported in the medical literature and in our own five patients, the urachal mucinous neoplasm presented the clinical picture of pseudomyxoma peritonei. The diagnosis of urachal mucinous adenocarcinoma is rarely made prior to the initial exploratory surgery; often, the necessary plans to definitively treat the disease are not formed. However, in the patient presented above, prior experience with this disease led to a diagnosis preoperatively, and definitive treatment with CRS and HIPEC occurred as a single event. The symptom of mucus noted upon urination should be recognized as an unusual complaint distinctively associated with this rare disease. Computed tomography showing a cystic mass anatomically related to the position of the urachus can also suggest the diagnosis. In some patients, this primary tumor mass may be noted prior to the development and progression of the extensive mucinous ascites described as pseudomyxoma peritonei. In our patient and others shown in Table 3.1, a greatly elevated CA 19-9 tumor marker was helpful in making a diagnosis of mucinous urachal PM and has been utilized in follow-up.

In patients who present with mucosuria and a cystic lower midline abdominal mass on CT or magnetic resonance imaging (MRI), a primary urachal adenocarcinoma should be suspected. During the prolonged course of this disease prior to diagnosis, the urachal mucinous neoplastic cells gain access to the peritoneal cavity. In this environment, they continue to disseminate as neoplastic cells in mucinous ascites moving with peritoneal fluid throughout the peritoneal cavity. This characteristic pattern of tumor dissemination associated with pseudomyxoma peritonei is known as "redistribution phenomenon" [2, 29]. In some patients, the mucus from the primary tumor mass is also forced down a patent urachus into the bladder, causing mucosuria. A definitive treatment approach to this disease using CRS and HIPEC similar to that used for patients with pseudomyxoma peritonei from an appendiceal mucinous neoplasm may be of greatest benefit to these patients.

Table 3.1 Literature review of urachal adenocarcinoma presenting with pseudomyxoma peritonei

Author	Year	N	Age/sex	Pathology	Cytoreduction	Cystectomy	HIPEC	Survival (months)	CEA/CA 19-9 preoperative	Current status
Mendeloff [7]	1971	1	49/M	Mucinous adenocarcinoma	Debulking	No	No	28	NA/NA	DOD
Sasano [19]	1997	1	45/M	Cystadenoma	None	No	No	NA	5.7/135	NA
Loggie [20]	1997	1	35/M	Signet ring	Extensive	Yes	Mitomycin C 40 mg	31	NA/NA	DOD
De Bree [12]	2000	1	34/M	Low-grade mucinous	Extensive	No	Mitomycin C	108	NA/NA	NED
Yanagisawa [21]	2003	1	50/F	Mucinous cystadenocarcinoma	Oophorectomy	No	No	NA	NA/NA	NED
Stenhouse [22]	2003	1	55/M	Low-grade mucinous	NA	No	No	NA	28/NA	NA
Takeuchi [23]	2004	1	82/M	Mucinous adenocarcinoma	Minimal	No	No	NA	7.9/38	NA
Sugarbaker [24]		4	32/F	Mucinous adenocarcinoma	Extensive	No	EPIC	132	4/182	DOD
			47/M	Mucinous adenocarcinoma	Extensive	No	Mitomycin C	20	14/594	NED
			51/M	Low-grade mucinosis	Extensive	No	No	68	NA/NA	DOD
			38/F	Adenocarcinoma	Extensive	No	Mitomycin C Doxorubicin	13	171/10	DOD
Shen [25]	2009	5	NA	NA	NA	NA	NA	NA	NA	NA
Glehen [26]	2010	4	NA	NA	NA	NA	NA	NA	NA	NA
Barrios [27]	2015	4	NA	NA	NA	NA	NA	NA	NA	NA
Sugarbaker [28]	2015	1	59/M	Adenomucinosis	Extensive	No	Cisplatin Doxorubicin Ifosfamide	10	15.6/94	NED

DOD died of disease, *HIPEC* hyperthermic intraperitoneal chemotherapy, *EPIC* early postoperative intraperitoneal chemotherapy using mitomycin C and 5-fluorouracil, *N* number of patients, *NA* not available, *NED* no evidence of disease, *units for CA 19-9* μ/mL, *units for CEA* ng/mL

3.2.4 Treatment of Urachal Pseudomyxoma Peritonei

Complete excision of a primary urachal adenocarcinoma with clear margins is the treatment of choice if primary cancer resection alone can achieve negative margins. The mucinous nature of this neoplasm and the possibility for stray cancer cells developing at a later time as pseudomyxoma peritonei must be considered. An en bloc resection of dome of the bladder and tumor is the preferred surgical strategy. The decision to proceed with a cystectomy versus simple resection of the superior aspect of the bladder with negative margins will depend on the anatomic extent of the disease and its biological aggressiveness. In the proper clinical setting, cystectomy is not mandatory [30]. In patients with pseudomyxoma peritonei arising in a primary urachal adenocarcinoma, the disease is associated with a cystic primary cancer that produces copious mucus. In this type of primary cancer, deep invasion into the bladder is less likely to occur. In our patients and in the others reported in the literature, cystectomy was not required. Although the primary urachal cancer is usually manageable by surgical resection, the peritoneal spread presents a special problem in management requiring CRS and HIPEC.

3.2.5 Follow-Up of Urachal Pseudomyxoma Peritonei

Most of these patients have an elevated CEA and CA 19-9 tumor marker at the time of diagnosis of the pseudomyxoma peritonei (Table 3.1). In our patients, the tumor markers increased with disease recurrence and declined to normal with CCRS. These tumor markers should be used in a serial manner in follow-up. These mucinous tumors are well imaged by CT, especially if the bowel is filled by oral contrast. We recommend for follow-up tumor markers CEA and CA 19-9 every 3 months and chest, abdominal, and pelvic CT every 6 months for 5 years post-cytoreduction. Similar recommendations have been made for appendiceal malignancies [31].

3.2.6 Pathology of Urachal Pseudomyxoma Peritonei

Urachal remnants are usually lined by transitional-type epithelium; however, focal glandular metaplasia may give rise to mucinous adenocarcinoma similar to that seen with colon cancer. These tumors are similar to appendiceal neoplasms in that there is a large spectrum of biological aggressiveness between patients. In some patients, the epithelial cells are described as bland, well differentiated, and non-invasive and are thought to be of borderline malignancy [22]. In other reports, an aggressive signet ring histomorphology is reported [19]. We have suggested that the term "mucinous urachal neoplasms" be used to describe this clinical entity to include this broad range of histologic types of noninvasive- as well as invasive-appearing tumors.

3.3 Pseudomyxoma Peritonei from Small Bowel Adenocarcinoma

3.3.1 Case Report

In January 1995, the patient developed intestinal obstruction. He was originally explored through an appendectomy incision and found to have mucinous small bowel adenocarcinoma. Through a midline incision, he underwent a right colon resection with resection of the primary colon in the terminal ileum. He was treated with six cycles of intraperitoneal 5-fluorouracil with systemic mitomycin C. He also had radiation therapy for progressive tumor within the appendectomy incision.

In January of 1996, the patient developed partial small bowel obstruction and was taken back to the operating room for excision of tumor from the abdominal wall with resection of the right rectus abdominis muscle and a redo right colon resection.

The patient did well for 2 years but then had recurrent small bowel obstruction, and in January 1998, he had a third resection. The patient was found to have extensive radiation fibrosis. An additional 3 ft of small bowel were removed along with resection of tumor in and along the right ureter. All specimens showed infiltrating metastatic mucinous adenocarcinoma. At the time of the third operation, the tumor had foci of poor differentiation with transmural involvement of the small bowel.

In February 1999, recurrent symptomatic tumor on the anterior abdominal wall was removed. In September 1999, hematuria developed and a cystoscopy showed mucinous adenocarcinoma infiltrating the wall of the bladder. Systemic chemotherapy and then best palliative care were initiated. The patient died in September 2000, 5 years and 9 months after his diagnosis.

3.3.2 Discussion

This patient demonstrates the gradual transition over time and with multiple interventions of tumor histology from low grade to higher grade. This change is associated with a less favorable outcome with repeated surgical interventions. The frequency of this change in the biology of a malignancy is not known but has been documented for pseudomyxoma peritonei of appendiceal origin [32].

Small bowel adenocarcinoma is a rare malignancy causing less than 5% of gastrointestinal cancer [33]. Only a fraction of small bowel adenocarcinoma patients will manifest pseudomyxoma peritonei. However, it does occur and can be successfully treated by CRS and HIPEC because of the relative sparing of the remainder of the small bowel by mucinous neoplasms [8]. The expected survival of small bowel adenocarcinoma with pseudomyxoma peritonei is not known. But a large multi-institutional experience with PM from small bowel adenocarcinoma is reported in the Monograph of the French Surgical Association [33]. They report on 45 patients who had a median survival of 32 months. The 1-, 3- and 5-year survival was 81%, 47%, and 33%, respectively. The clinical factors influencing survival were the experience of the institution treating the patient ($p = 0.048$) and the completeness of cytoreduction ($p \leq 0.001$). The number of patients with mucinous peritoneal metastases in this experience was not reported.

Evaluation of this data regarding the efficacy of CRS and HIPEC is difficult because there is little or no information regarding the survival of patients with PM from small bowel cancer treated by surgery alone. Fishman et al. have reported the largest series treated with chemotherapy demonstrating a 30% response rate. The use of palliative chemotherapy in this setting of metastatic and locally advanced unresectable disease achieved a median survival of 11 months [34]. Currently, combinations of systemic chemotherapy combined with CRS and perioperative chemotherapy can be recommended in patients having mucinous peritoneal metastases from small bowel adenocarcinoma with a moderate to low PCI and the possibility of a complete cytoreduction.

3.4   Mesenteric Cyst Resulting in Pseudomyxoma Peritonei

3.4.1   Case Report

A 38-year-old woman was presented in June 2008 with diffuse mucinous ascites with intra-abdominal and pelvic neoplasm. Her initial symptoms of fatigue, urinary frequency, fever, weight gain, and moderate abdominal pain began after her pregnancy in 2003. The symptoms became more severe in December 2007, with increased abdominal fullness and pain. She sought medical advice and a diagnosis of pelvic inflammation was made. The antibiotic treatment she underwent was not helpful. A CT scan was performed which showed mucoid ascites in the abdomen and pelvis. An exploratory laparotomy was performed in January 2008. Mucoid ascitic fluid was drained during the surgical intervention. Copious mucoid tumor was found on the peritoneal surfaces, especially involving the greater and lesser omentum. A total abdominal hysterectomy, bilateral salpingo-oophorectomy, mesenteric cystectomy, omentectomy, and appendectomy were performed. A large mesenteric cyst was resected and is shown in Fig. 3.6a, b.

Because of uncertainty regarding the etiology of the primary tumor, the pathology specimens were sent to other medical centers for review. An ovarian teratoma present in the resected specimen was not considered to be the primary site because it did not contain epithelium or mucinous material. However, the ruptured mesenteric cyst contained abundant borderline neoplastic mucinous epithelium. The diagnosis was pseudomyxoma peritonei originating from malignant transformation of a mesenteric cyst.

At our institution, the CT scan revealed residual mucinous tumor nodules at multiple sites within the abdomen and pelvis. Persistent tumor was layered out beneath the right hemidiaphragm, class 0 changes were present within the small bowel mesentery, and a mass had developed at the apex of the vagina.

The patient underwent a complete CRS followed by HIPEC plus 5-fluorouracil. Mitomycin C and doxorubicin were given by the intraperitoneal route and 5-fluorouracil and leucovorin by intravenous administration [35]. The pathology returned as disseminated peritoneal adenomucinosis (DPAM) (Fig. 3.7). The decision

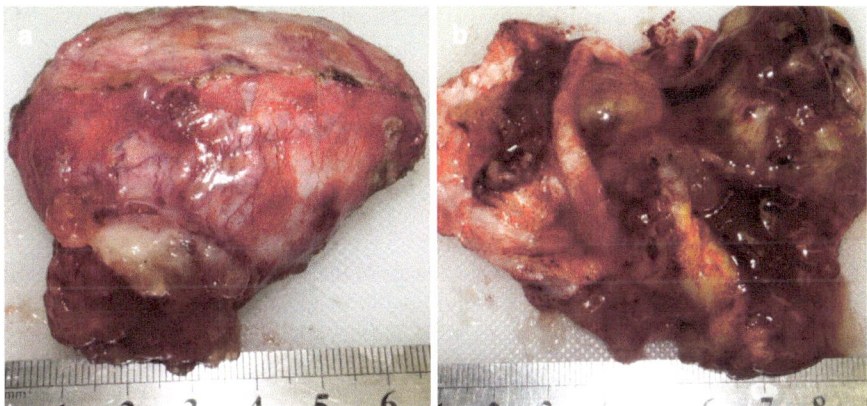

Fig. 3.6 Photograph of the mesenteric cyst removed at initial surgical intervention. (**a**) The cyst was perforated with mucus extruding from its surface. (**b**) The cyst was bisected to show its multilocular character and mucinous contents (From Sugarbaker [59], with permission)

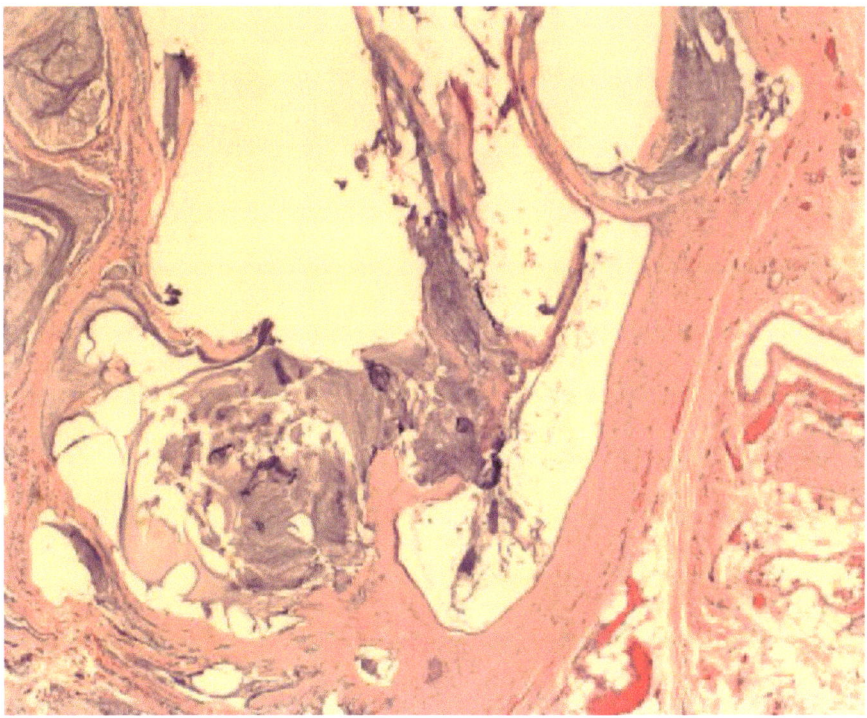

Fig. 3.7 Photomicrograph of tumor in a patient with a mesenteric cyst taken from the pelvis showed adenomucinosis. The peritoneal lesions showed simple mucinous epithelial strips with abundant extracellular mucin. Bland epithelium had no cytological atypia or mitosis (hematoxylin and eosin ×500) (From Sugarbaker [59], with permission)

was made not to recommend any further treatment. The patient is asymptomatic and on a 6-monthly CT scan regimen for the next 5 years. She remains well with no evidence of disease at 6 years.

3.4.2 Discussion

Mesenteric cysts can be seen within the leaves of the mesentery from the duodenum to the rectum and may be single or multilocular. The small bowel mesentery (50%) is the most frequent location, followed by the mesocolon (33%) and mesorectum (10%). The contents of the cyst may be mucinous, serous, chylous, bloody, or mixed. A majority presents with cuboidal or columnar epithelial lining with a lack of atypical morphology. Although unusual, malignant transformation of a mesenteric cyst may occur. In an extensive literature review by O'Brien et al., malignant transformation was described in four cases [36].

Our patient with pseudomyxoma peritonei arising from a ruptured mesenteric cyst was treated with CRS and perioperative chemotherapy. This treatment plan has been used extensively for the curative approach to pseudomyxoma peritonei of appendiceal origin [31]. The majority of mucinous appendiceal neoplasms are perforated at the time of diagnosis, and copious mucinous ascites with the pseudomyxoma peritonei are evident. The CRS procedure combined with HIPEC has resulted in long-term survival in a majority of these patients. By analogy, this treatment for pseudomyxoma peritonei of appendiceal origin was applied in the patient described in this report.

Although the etiology of mesenteric cysts is poorly defined and its ideal management has yet to be determined, ultrasound is the preferred imaging tool at the initial stages of investigation [37]. Computed tomography scan and MRI are helpful for its localization and anatomical definition. Complete excision is the goal of treatment and should be extended to the attached bowel, if necessary. If the cyst has ruptured and is extruding mucus-containing epithelial cells, a diagnosis of pseudomyxoma peritonei must be considered. In these patients, in addition to excision of the primary tumor, CRS and perioperative chemotherapy should be a standard of care.

3.5 Tailgut Cyst as a Cause of Pseudomyxoma Peritonei

3.5.1 Case Report

In December 2005, a 37-year-old woman was presented with abdominal discomfort, vaginal bleeding, and rectal fullness of 2-year duration. Intravaginal ultrasonography and abdominal MRI were performed and revealed an ill-defined complex mass on the left side of the pelvis measuring 6.5×3.6 cm. The mass was thick walled and had a prominent cystic component. The left ovary and uterus were uninvolved.

She underwent a local resection of a left-sided presacral tumor mass, appendectomy, and left oophorectomy. The pathology report showed a well-differentiated mucinous adenocarcinoma arising in a retrorectal hamartoma. The appendix and left ovary were not involved and were excluded as primary sites. The piecemeal resection of the primary tumor mass was thought to be complete, but the resection was not en bloc. Because of the possibility of persistent disease and the absence of further treatment options at the outside institution, systemic chemotherapy was recommended. The patient was started on a systemic chemotherapy regimen including oxaliplatin, 5-fluorouracil, and Avastin. The treatment was followed by capecitabine and carboplatin.

In March 2007, disease progression was documented by computed tomography (CT) scan. She underwent a CT-guided biopsy of an omental nodule which confirmed the presence of mucinous adenocarcinoma. Additional systemic chemotherapy with cisplatin and paclitaxel was administered at the outside institution because no other treatment options were considered appropriate.

Repeat CT performed in September 2007 showed mucinous tumor nodules located within the greater omentum, and a complex mucinous mass consisting of sigmoid colon, uterus, right ovary, and tumor filled the pelvis (Figs. 3.8 and 3.9). The radiological findings were consistent with a high-grade pseudomyxoma peritonei disseminated within the abdomen and pelvis.

Cytoreductive surgery was performed in September 2007 and included a total abdominal hysterectomy, bilateral salpingectomy, right oophorectomy, greater omentectomy, lesser omentectomy, pelvic peritonectomy, splenectomy, and left ureterolysis. Following optimal cytoreduction, HIPEC utilizing intraperitoneal mitomycin C and doxorubicin plus systemic 5-fluorouracil and leucovorin were administered at 42 °C. The selection of this combination of chemotherapy for this rare disease was based on pharmacological studies [35].

The histological findings were compatible with mucinous PM with intermediate features (Fig. 3.10). Extracellular mucin pools were associated with mildly atypical simple mucinous epithelium and focally stratified epithelium with moderate atypia.

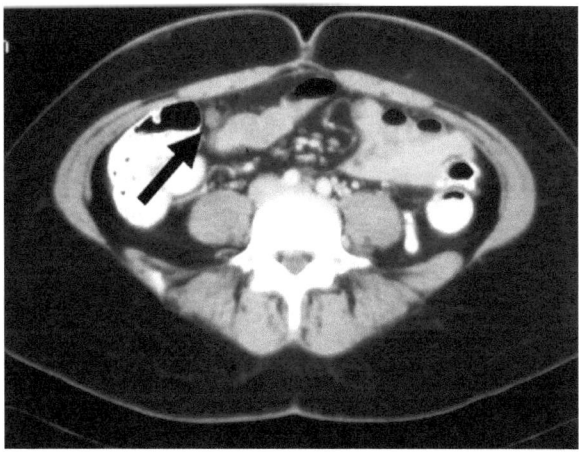

Fig. 3.8 CT scan in a patient with pararectal hamartoma through the mid-abdomen showing recurrent mucinous tumor involving the greater omentum. CT-guided biopsy of this omental mass showed adenocarcinoma. The mass is indicated by an *arrow* (From Sugarbaker [59], with permission)

Fig. 3.9 CT scan in a patient with pararectal hamartoma through the pelvis showing a complex mass consisting of sigmoid colon, uterus, ovaries, and mucinous tumor recurrent at the site of primary tumor resection. The predominant tumor mass is indicated by an *arrow* (From Sugarbaker [59], with permission)

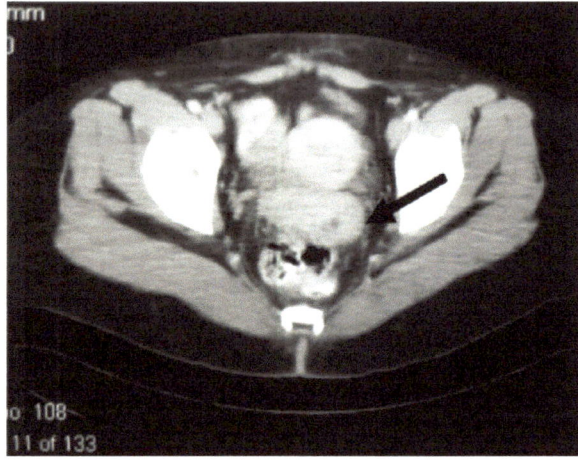

Fig. 3.10 Histological findings in a patient with tailgut cyst of pseudomyxoma peritonei with intermediate features. Small areas of focally stratified epithelium that is moderately pleomorphic suggested an intermediate type of peritoneal mucinous carcinoma. A great majority of the resected specimen was acellular mucus (hematoxylin and eosin ×400). (From Sugarbaker [59], with permission)

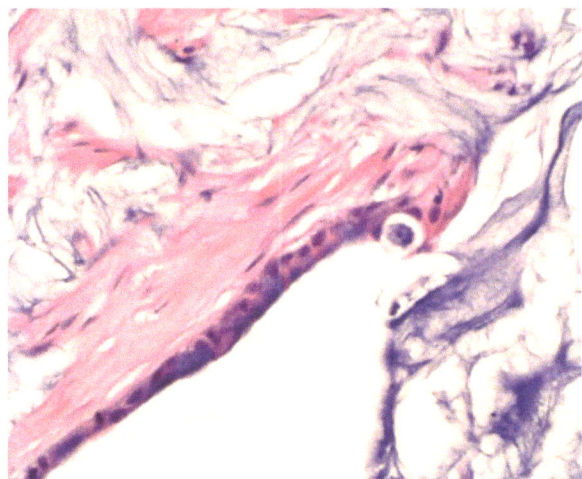

Immunohistochemical studies were not performed. The right ovary was normal. The hospital course was uneventful, and the patient was discharged home on her 15th hospital day. As of April of 2011, the patient was alive with local recurrence invading the sacrum. The peritoneal cavity has remained free of disease. Attempts at local excision of the sacral mass with cryosurgical treatment of the margins of excision were unsuccessful. The patient has received palliative external beam radiotherapy.

3.5.2   Discussion

Tailgut cyst or retrorectal hamartoma is a rare congenital lesion. It is believed to originate from the remnant of the tailgut, which is a primitive gut temporarily present at the caudal portion of the embryo. The tailgut atrophies disappear completely at an adult age. However, if vestigial remnants persist, these can be the origin of a retrorectal hamartoma. These cysts are lined with different epithelium types that may be found in the embryological gastrointestinal tract, including stratified squamous, ciliated columnar, mucin-secreting columnar, and transitional-type epithelium [38–40]. Tailgut cysts can occur at any age but are seen predominantly in middle-aged women. The female to male ratio is 3:1.

Malignant transformations, including development of adenocarcinoma or carcinoid, are known to occur in retrorectal hamartomas. The incidence of this malignant transformation is not available from the surgical literature, but it is assumed to be rare. The adenocarcinomas are usually moderately to poorly differentiated and strongly positive for carcinoembryonic antigen [40]. The possibility of malignant degeneration of the otherwise benign-appearing cyst defines the need for complete surgical excision of the mass in the absence of tumor spillage.

The definitive treatment of the primary tailgut cyst is complete surgical excision; this may include en bloc resection of a portion of the rectum. Preoperative biopsy should not be attempted because of the risk of spreading dysplastic cells through a punctured cyst wall. If the mass is surgically unresectable at presentation, incisional biopsy can be attempted, but the surgeon should be aware that this approach may result in mucinous cancer dissemination.

Very rarely does a tailgut cyst spontaneously rupture into the peritoneal cavity. Local recurrences do occur after incomplete excision and spillage of cancer cells. This may result from the trauma of surgical excision causing implantation at the resection site and widespread mucinous PM. In our patient, a large mass of mucinous cancer to the left of the rectum was removed "piecemeal" along with an extensive amount of mucinous tumor within the presacral region. This progression of a large volume of pseudomyxoma peritonei within the free peritoneal cavity occurred as a result of surgical trauma with resection of the primary tumor mass. Because of the intermediate invasive nature of this malignancy, at the time of CRS, optimal resection of the disease that was disseminated within the abdomen and pelvis was possible. Microscopic disease that may have remained in the peritoneal cavity following cytoreduction was treated with HIPEC.

Unfortunately, residual tumor along the left side of the rectum was contained in the scar tissue that was associated with the primary tumor resection and was not included as a rectal resection with CRS. It was not eradicated by perioperative chemotherapy. The tumor was deeply invasive into the upper sacrum at the time of recurrence after CRS and perioperative chemotherapy. Similarly, rectal cancer recurrent after low-anterior resection or abdominoperineal resection with PM is rarely benefitted by CRS and HIPEC as a result of progression of pelvic cancer seeding [41].

To our knowledge, this is the first case of pseudomyxoma peritonei reported in the medical literature that had a retrorectal hamartoma origin. Pseudomyxoma peritonei most frequently arises from a ruptured appendiceal adenoma and progresses with a large volume of mucinous tumor distributed throughout the abdomen and pelvis in a characteristic fashion. The standard of care for this disease is complete cytoreduction using visceral resections and peritonectomy procedures combined with HIPEC in an attempt to eradicate gross and microscopic disease [42, 43].

3.6 Pseudomyxoma Peritonei Arising from Spilled Tumor Cells with Resection of the Colon or Rectal Polyps

3.6.1 Case Report

A 71-year-old woman underwent surgery to remove a large tubulovillous adenoma of the rectum. After resection of the rectosigmoid colon, examination of the specimen did not show the expected tumor mass. The adenoma was determined to be within the residual rectum. At the same operative procedure, a more extensive rectal resection was performed, and the tubulovillous adenoma was adequately resected at this time. Postoperative microscopic exam showed a rectal villous adenoma with dysplastic changes.

Three years later during a hernia repair, the surgeon observed mucous ascites coming from the peritoneal cavity. A few weeks later, the patient underwent a major debulking procedure. One year later, the CT showed tumor around the liver and another mass occupying the left side of her abdomen going down to fill the pelvis. She was referred to our service and underwent CRS followed by HIPEC with mitomycin C chemotherapy. Histopathology showed DPAM with areas of atypia. The pseudomyxoma peritonei was thought to arise from the spillage of tumor cells at the time the sigmoid colon polyp was removed 4 years prior. She remains disease-free after 3 years' follow-up.

The first report of pseudomyxoma arising from colonic polyps was by Goldstein et al. who presented three patients with a colorectal polyp as the origin for pseudomyxoma peritonei [14]. As a result of copious mucus production, cells from these neoplasms spread throughout the peritoneal cavity with the same efficiency as a ruptured appendiceal adenoma. This case report demonstrates that when the surgeon performs an open resection of colonic polyps, great care should be taken to avoid spillage of dysplastic cells which may result in iatrogenic development of pseudomyxoma peritonei.

3.7 Pseudomyxoma Peritonei from Peritoneal Dissemination of an Ovarian Malignancy of Low Malignant Potential

In April 2002, a 34-year-old woman had a debulking procedure through a Pfannenstiel incision. The diagnosis was mucinous cystadenoma of ovarian origin. Almost immediately postoperatively, tumor progression was noted. She had multiple paracenteses to remove fluid from the peritoneal cavity. Symptoms progressed until urinary and gastrointestinal functions were seriously compromised.

In September 2004, with complaints of massively distended abdomen, absence of urinary function, and near-complete bowel obstruction, the patient was seen at MedStar Washington Hospital Center. She underwent an 8-h cytoreduction with hysterectomy and bilateral salpingo-oophorectomy, left colectomy with low anastomosis and pelvic peritonectomy. She was treated with HIPEC using cisplatin (5 mg/m^2) and doxorubicin (15 mg/m^2). At 10 years' follow-up, the patient remains disease-free.

3.7.1 Discussion

To date, our service has treated three patients with extensive PM from mucinous ovarian malignancy. All three patients had large masses within the pelvis that resulted in ureteral obstruction. In the patient presented, both bilateral ureteral obstruction and sigmoid colon obstruction had occurred. The three patients remain free of disease at 7, 10, and 14 years postoperatively.

3.8 Pseudomyxoma Peritonei from Mucinous Endocervical Cancer

A 33-year-old woman with morbid obesity on a weight-loss program continued to gain weight. Her only pertinent history was a cone biopsy for cervical dysplasia performed in 2002. No invasive malignancy could be documented. Because of pain, she went to an emergency room where ultrasound showed a large amount of ascites with solid tumor in the pelvis. In May 2011, a paracentesis for 5 l of serous and mucinous ascites was performed. Cytology on the fluid was negative. Two weeks later, she was taken back to the operating room for a laparoscopy. Bilateral ovarian masses were visualized and biopsies taken. An additional 9 l of ascites were removed. One month later, 12 l of ascites were removed under CT control (Figs. 3.11 and

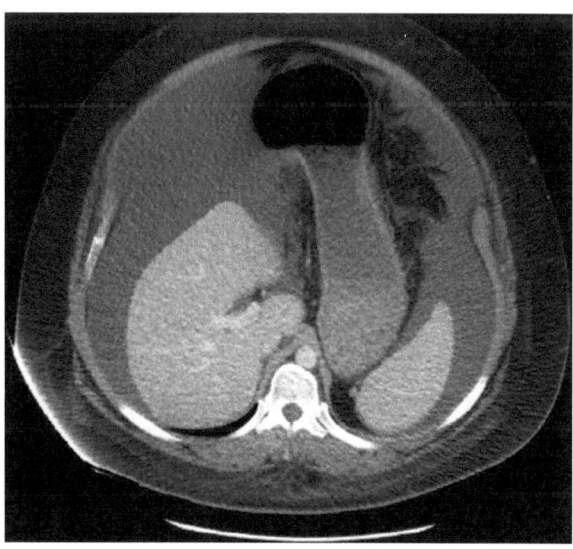

Fig. 3.11 CT through the upper abdomen in a patient with debilitating ascites from cervical adenocarcinoma (From Sugarbaker [59], with permission)

Fig. 3.12 CT through the mid-abdomen in a patient with debilitating ascites from adenocarcinoma of the cervix. The serous ascites is extensive. The small bowel is compartmentalized within the mid-abdomen and shows no evidence of dysfunction (From Sugarbaker [59], with permission)

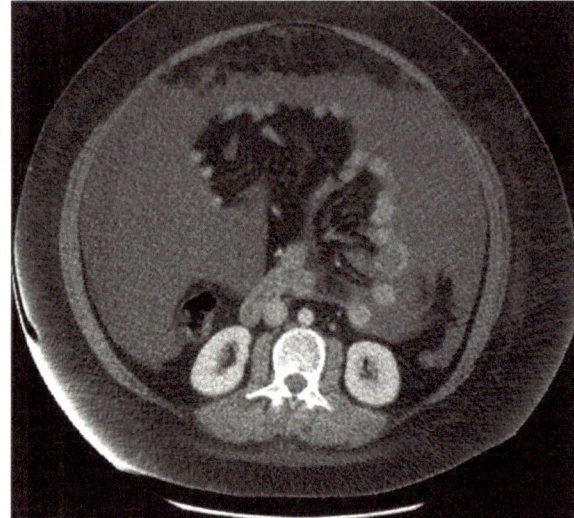

Fig. 3.13 Intraoperative photograph of a patient with peritoneal metastases from adenocarcinoma of the cervix. Peritoneal surfaces in the right upper quadrant and pelvis were layered by the mucinous tumor. Both the right and left ovaries showed large mucinous metastases. The loops of the small bowel seen in the foreground of this photo are free of mucinous tumor (From Sugarbaker [59], with permission)

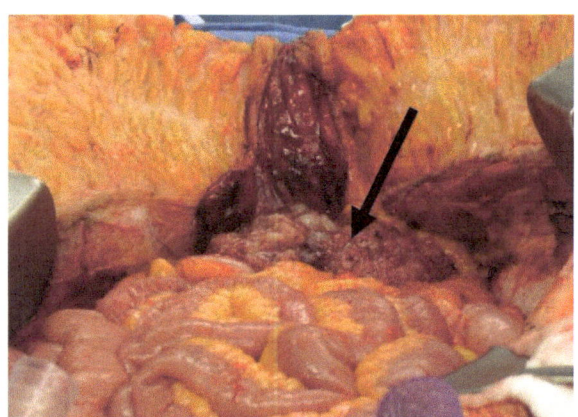

3.12). A preoperative colonoscopy was negative. In July 2011, the patient underwent a 9-h CRS procedure. Peritonectomy of the right upper quadrant and pelvis was required along with hysterectomy and removal of large ovarian masses (Fig. 3.13). After the CRS, HIPEC with doxorubicin and cisplatin plus systemic ifosfamide plus mesna were used. Postoperatively, the patient developed a wound infection treated by conservative measures.

Pathology of the hysterectomy specimen showed an in situ and invasive mucinous adenocarcinoma of the endocervix. The cervical stromal invasion was superficial despite examination of the cervix in its entirety. All of the specimens from abdominal and pelvic surfaces showed metastatic mucinous adenocarcinoma consistent with a primary endocervical adenocarcinoma.

3.8.1 Discussion

To our knowledge, this is the first patient with pseudomyxoma peritonei from a mucinous endocervical cancer who has been treated with CRS and HIPEC. Data regarding the long-term benefits from this approach had not yet been established. This patient has remained with no evidence of disease progression at 5 years.

The pathophysiology of cervical adenocarcinoma dissemination to the peritoneal surfaces is not readily apparent. Recently, retrograde menstruation from the fallopian tubes has been suggested to cause what was previously identified as serous ovarian cancer [44]. It is possible that adenocarcinoma cells from the endocervix could likewise, in unusual patients, spread into the free peritoneal space through a process of retrograde menstruation. Two of our three patients were young and nulliparous. These are the patients who are most likely to develop endometriosis, which is a manifestation of normal endometrial tissue entering the peritoneal space through the process of retrograde menstruation. Also, in all three of our patients, there was extensive mucus and serous fluid produced by the malignancy leading to profound abdominal distention in all three patients. The demonstrated ability of endocervical adenocarcinoma to produce such copious amounts of fluid seems well documented by our three patients. Copious slippery fluid discharged into the uterus may be forced into the fallopian tubes and be expressed into the free peritoneal space. Of course, the fluid would be contaminated by mucinous cancer cells and would soon lead to the extensive mucinous ascites and peritoneal metastases present in our patients.

Uterine perforation can result in direct inoculation of cancer cells into the free peritoneal space. Anecdotal reports from the gynecologic oncology literature document this fact. In 1981, Mills, Sugg, and Mahnesmith reported the direct extension of a uterine adenosarcoma through the wall of the uterus and growing out as a pelvic mass attached to the uterine serosa [45]. The cancer inside and outside of the uterus was histologically identical. They identified this clinical situation as the first reported example of direct inoculation of a cancer into the peritoneal space following myometrial perforation. Levine et al. noted trophoblastic tissue spread to the surface of the sigmoid colon following uterine perforation during dilatation and curettage. A laparotomy showed trophoblastic tumor implants at the perforation site, anterior uterine wall, and appendix epiploica of the sigmoid colon. Surgical removal and treatment with methotrexate enabled the patient to recover [46]. A possible mechanism of dissemination of endocervical adenocarcinoma into the free peritoneal cavity would be uterine perforation at the time of a cervical dilatation and curettage. However, no surgical record of uterine perforation was present in our patients, and the patients were not aware that such an event had occurred.

The applications of CRS and HIPEC have been evolving and expanding over the last 30 years. This combined treatment has been shown to be of benefit in the management of intraabdominal malignancies, especially those having a high propensity for peritoneal metastases [47]. To our knowledge, this is the first report of CRS and HIPEC for endocervical adenocarcinoma with ovarian and peritoneal metastases with the pseudomyxoma peritonei syndrome [48]. Further clinical studies are required to assess the durability of this approach to this unusual manifestation of endocervical adenocarcinoma.

3.9   The Use of Quantitative Prognostic Indicators to Select Patients for CRS and HIPEC

Pseudomyxoma peritonei is the clinical description of a low to moderate grade mucinous neoplasm with peritoneal dissemination. These neoplasms are the paradigm by which the principles of the management of peritoneal surface malignancy have evolved. A large proportion but, as documented in this book chapter, not all of these conditions originate in the appendix.

The evaluation of patients using a series of prognostic indicators reliably used to select patients for CRS and HIPEC include (1) an estimate of the biological aggressiveness of the malignant process through histopathologic assessment [3, 49], (2) use of preoperative CT scan to exclude patients with confluence of disease associated with the small bowel [50–52], (3) estimates of the extent of disease through use of the peritoneal cancer index (PCI), and (4) determination of the completeness of cytoreduction (CC) score at the conclusion of the peritonectomy procedures and visceral resections [31, 53].

These principles of management not only apply to appendiceal malignancy, but they have also been used to more knowledgeably select patients with pseudomyxoma from non-appendiceal sites [54, 55]. With validation of these quantitative prognostic indicators in a large number of malignancies associated with peritoneal dissemination, it may be possible to select patients with unusual abdominal and pelvic neoplasms that have PM for successful treatment by CRS and perioperative chemotherapy.

A summary of the clinical data for the use of quantitative prognostic indicators is as follows: Patient selection is restricted to those with a low PCI (<10) if the malignancy is of an aggressive nature. For example, colorectal PM treated in patients with PCI ≤10 is expected to show a 50% long-term benefit from treatment. Patients with a PCI >20 rarely achieve more than palliative benefit [56]. In contrast, patients with low biological grade of malignancy can benefit if the CRS is complete despite very high PCI. For example, Sugarbaker showed that patients who had an appendiceal mucinous neoplasm with adenomucinosis and a PCI >20 had a 20-year survival of 65% [31]. There is a strong rationale that supports CRS and perioperative chemotherapy as a valid treatment option to be considered in patients with pseudomyxoma peritonei. Because of small bowel sparing and a noninvasive tumor biology, a PCI often >20, complete CRS, and long-term, disease-free survival have been documented. The results of treatment are in sharp contrast to those for PM from colon and rectal cancer or from gastric cancer, where treatment benefits are small with a PCI >20 even if cytoreduction is complete [47]. For appendiceal or non-appendiceal pseudomyxoma peritonei, the results of treatment are similar. Long-term survival is possible with a complete cytoreduction even though the PCI is >20 [31].

The recent publications of Kalluri and Weinberg may provide a molecular basis for our results [57]. The hypothesis of epithelial-mesenchymal transition states that the aggressive biology of a carcinoma to an invasive and metastatic potential develops along with a fibrotic matrix. The growth factors that control this malignant transition are produced by transformed stem cells; the more plentiful the stem cells are, the greater the extent of the fibrous stroma. This fibrotic response results in a marked increase in chemotherapy resistance. The stem cells have increased intrinsic chemotherapy resistance, and the fibrosis interferes with chemotherapy access to cancer cells.

In many of the diseases presented in this book chapter, the epithelial to mesenchymal transition had not yet begun to express itself. The epithelial character of the malignancy was preserved, and a fibrous stroma was minimal facilitating a complete cytoreduction. The prediction of a chemotherapy response of residual cancer cells after CRS would be supported by the Weinberg model. In summary, an absence of epithelial to mesenchymal transition would indicate a high likelihood of benefit from CRS and HIPEC.

3.10   Early Referral of Rare Causes of Pseudomyxoma Peritonei Indicated

In most of the patients presented in this chapter, a large extent of disease was documented, and patients were referred to our service as they became symptomatic late in the natural history of the disease. This clinical situation required a lengthy CRS with a large number of visceral resections and peritonectomy procedures, which in turn requires a long hospital course and an extended period of recovery after hospital discharge. This extensive CRS may be avoidable. These patients often have clinical findings that suggest a high likelihood of progression of peritoneal surface malignancy at the time of their primary tumor excision. Perforation of the primary tumor, tumor rupture prior to or at the time of resection, ovarian Krukenberg-type metastases, and positive cytology are indications of a high likelihood of peritoneal surface progression of the neoplasm. Treatment at the time of primary cancer resection at a peritoneal surface oncology center would be the ideal management strategy. However, because these diseases are unusual, recommendation of a second look surgery 6–12 months postoperatively in a search for residual PM is an option in management [58]. Treatment of a large volume of disease with a high PCI (>20) is the least favorable treatment option for these patients.

Although the number of patients with non-appendiceal pseudomyxoma peritonei is small, the implications of success documented in these patient presentations may be quite meaningful. In the absence of special treatments, patients with pseudomyxoma peritonei from all diseases have a uniformly lethal outcome. The progression of the disease may be indolent, but the end result is always a terminal condition. Inclusion of CRS and HIPEC as an option should be considered as an addition to the treatments of these patients.

This collection of non-appendiceal pseudomyxoma peritonei treated by CRS and HIPEC should not be considered as comprehensive. There are undoubtedly other malignancies that have not undergone the epithelial to mesenchymal transition that are candidates for these treatments. The experienced peritoneal surface oncology center should be aware of the benefits offered by CRS and HIPEC for selected patients and be willing to consider these treatments as options for this group of patients.

References

1. Fann JI, Vierra M, Fisher D, Oberhelman HA, Cobb L. Pseudomyxoma peritonei. Surg Gynecol Obstet. 1993;177:441–7.
2. Carmignani P, Sugarbaker TA, Bromley CM, Sugarbaker PH. Intraperitoneal cancer dissemination: mechanisms of the patterns of spread. Cancer Metastasis Rev. 2003;22:465–72.
3. Ronnett BM, Zahn CM, Kurman RJ, et al. Disseminated peritoneal adenomucinosis and peritoneal mucinous carcinomatosis: a clinicopathologic analysis of 109 cases with emphasis on distinguishing pathologic features, site of origin, prognosis, and relationship to "pseudomyxoma peritonei". Am J Surg Pathol. 1995;19:1390–408.
4. Chejfec G, Rieker WJ, Jablokow VR, Gould VE. Pseudomyxoma peritonei associated with colloid carcinoma of the pancreas. Gastroenterology. 1986;90:202–5.
5. Zanelli M, Casadei R, Santini D, et al. Pseudomyxoma peritonei associated with intraductal papillary-mucinous neoplasm of the pancreas. Pancreas. 1998;17:100–2.
6. Honore C, Goere D, Dartigues P, et al. Peritoneal carcinomatosis from solid pseudopapillary neoplasm (Frantz's tumour) of the pancreas treated with HIPEC. Anticancer Res. 2012;32:1069–74.
7. Mendeloff J, McSwain Jr NE. Pseudomyxoma peritonei due to mucinous adenocarcinoma of the urachus. South Med J. 1971;64:497–8.
8. Marchettini P, Sugarbaker PH. Mucinous adenocarcinoma of the small bowel with peritoneal seeding. Case report and review of the literature. Eur J Surg Oncol. 2002;28:19–23.
9. Young RH, Scully RE. Ovarian metastasis from carcinoma of the gallbladder and extrahepatic bile ducts simulating primary tumor of ovary. A report of six cases. Int J Gynecol Pathol. 1990;9:60–72.
10. McCarthy JH, Aga R. A fallopian tube lesion of borderline malignancy associated with pseudomyxoma peritonei. Histopathology. 1988;12:223–5.
11. Ikejiri K, Anai H, Kitamura K, Yakabe S, Saku M, Yoshida K. Pseudomyxoma peritonei concomitant with early gastric cancer: report of a case. Surg Today. 1996;26:923–5.
12. de Bree E, Witkamp A, Van de Vijver M, Zoetmulder F. Unusual origins of pseudomyxoma peritonei. J Surg Oncol. 2000;75:270–4.
13. Ng WC, Yeoh SC, Joseph VT, Ong BH. Adenomyoma of the pylorus presenting as intestinal obstruction with pseudomyxoma peritonei – a case report. Ann Acad Med. 1981;10:562–5.
14. Goldstein PJ, Cabanas J, da Silva RG, Sugarbaker PH. Pseudomyxoma peritonei arising from colonic polyps. Eur J Surg Oncol. 2006;32:764–6.
15. Kurita M, Komatsu H, Hata Y, et al. Pseudomyxoma peritonei due to adenocarcinoma of the lung: case report. J Gastroenterol. 1994;29:344–8.
16. Hawes D, Robinson R, Wira R. Pseudomyxoma peritonei from metastatic colloid carcinoma of the breast. Gastrointest Radiol. 1991;16:80–2.
17. Zanarini D, Sugarbaker PH. Extremity soft tissue sarcoma with metastases to abdomino-pelvic surfaces. J Surg Oncol. 1997;64:68–73.
18. Sugarbaker PH. Peritonectomy procedures. Surg Oncol Clin N Am. 2003;12:703–27.
19. Sugarbaker PH. An overview of peritonectomy, visceral resections, and perioperative chemotherapy for peritoneal surface malignancy. In: Sugarbaker PH, editor. Cytoreductive surgery

& perioperative chemotherapy for peritoneal surface malignancy. Textbook and video atlas. Woodbury: Cine-Med Publishing; 2012. p. 1–30.
20. Loggie BW, Fleming RA, Hosseinian AA. Peritoneal carcinomatosis with urachal signet-cell adenocarcinoma. Urology. 1997;50:446–8.
21. Yanagisawa S, Fujinaga Y, Kadoya M. Urachal mucinous cystadenocarcinoma with a cystic ovarian metastasis. Am J Roentgenol. 2003;180:1183–5.
22. Stenhouse G, McRae D, Pollock AM. Urachal adenocarcinoma in situ with pseudomyxoma peritonei: a case report. J Clin Pathol. 2003;56:152–3.
23. Takeuchi M, Matsuzaki K, Yoshida S, et al. Imaging findings of urachal mucinous cystadeno-carcinoma associated with pseudomyxoma peritonei. Acta Radiol. 2004;45:348–50.
24. Sugarbaker PH, Verghese M, Yan TD, Brun E. Management of mucinous urachal neoplasm presenting as pseudomyxoma peritonei. Tumori. 2008;94:732–6.
25. Shen P, Stewart 4th JH, Levine EA. Cytoreductive surgery and intraperitoneal hyperther-mic chemotherapy for peritoneal surface malignancy: non colorectal indications. Curr Probl Cancer. 2009;33:168–93.
26. Glehen O, Osinski D, Baujard AL, Gilly PM. Natural history of peritoneal carcinomatosis from non gynecological malignancies. Surg Oncol N Am. 2003;12:720–39.
27. Barrios P. Barcelona, Spain. Personal communication.
28. Sugarbaker PH. Washington, DC. Unpublished data.
29. Sugarbaker PH. Pseudomyxoma peritonei: a cancer whose biology is characterized by a redis-tribution phenomenon. Ann Surg. 1994;219:109–11.
30. Santucci RA, True LD, Lange PH. Is partial cystectomy the treatment of choice for mucinous adenocarcinoma of the urachus? Urology. 1997;49:536–40.
31. Sugarbaker PH. Epithelial appendiceal neoplasms. Cancer J. 2009;15:225–35.
32. Yan H, Pestieau SR, Shmookler BM, Sugarbaker PH. Histopathologic analysis in 46 patients with pseudomyxoma peritonei syndrome: failure vs. success with a second-look operation. Mod Pathol. 2001;14(3):164–71.
33. Glehen O, Elias D, Gilly FN. Presentation du rapport de l'Association Francaise de Chirurgie. In: Elias D, Gilly FN, Glehen O, editors. Carcinoses Peritoneales D'Origine Digestive et Primitive. France: Arnette Wolkers Kluwer; 2008. p. 101–52.
34. Fishman PN, Pond GR, Moore MJ, et al. Natural history and chemotherapy effectiveness for advanced adenocarcinoma of the small bowel: a retrospective review of 113 cases. Am J Clin Oncol. 2006;29:225–31.
35. Van der Speeten K, Stuart OA, Sugarbaker PH. Pharmacokinetics and pharmacody-namics of perioperative cancer chemotherapy in peritoneal surface malignancy. Cancer J. 2009;15:216–24.
36. O'Brien MF, Winter DC, Lee G, Fitzgerald EJ, O'Sullivan GC. Mesenteric cysts. A series of six cases with a review of the literature. Ir J Med Sci. 1999;168:233–6.
37. de Perrot M, Brundler MA, Totsch M, Mentha G, Morel P. Mesenteric cysts. Towards less confusion? Dig Surg. 2000;17:323–8.
38. Costello D, Schofield A, Stirling R, Theodorou N. Extrarectal mass: a tailgut cyst. J R Soc Med. 2000;93:85–6.
39. Killingsworth C, Gadacz T. Tailgut cyst (retrorectal hamartoma): report of a case and review of literature. Am Surg. 2005;71:666–71.
40. Kantham SC, Kanthan R. Unusual retrorectal lesion. Asian J Surg. 2004;27:144–6.
41. da Silva RG, Sugarbaker PH. Analysis of prognostic factors in seventy patients having a com-plete cytoreduction plus perioperative intraperitoneal chemotherapy for carcinomatosis from colorectal cancer. J Am Coll Surg. 2006;203:878–86.
42. Sugarbaker PH, Ronnett BM, Archer A, et al. Pseudomyxoma peritonei syndrome. Adv Surg. 1996;30:233–80.
43. Sugarbaker PH. New standard of care for appendiceal epithelial malignancies and pseudo-myxoma peritonei syndrome. Lancet Oncol. 2006;7:69–76.
44. Kurman RJ, Shih IM. Molecular pathogenesis and extraovarian origin of epithelial ovarian cancer – shifting the paradigm. Hum Pathol. 2011;42:918–31.

45. Mills SE, Sugg NK, Mahnesmith RC. Endometrial adenosarcoma with pelvic involvement following uterine perforation. Diagn Gynecol Obstet. 1981;3:149–54.
46. Levin I, Grisaru D, Pauzner D, Almog B. Trophoblastic tissue spread to the sigmoid colon after uterine perforation. Obstet Gynecol. 2004;104:1172–4.
47. Glehen O, Gilly FN, Boutitie F, et al. Toward curative treatment of peritoneal carcinomatosis from nonovarian origin by cytoreductive surgery combined with perioperative intraperitoneal chemotherapy: a multi-institutional study of 1,200 patients. Cancer. 2010;116:5608–18.
48. Sugarbaker PH, Rangole A, Carr NJ. Peritoneal metastases from mucinous endocervical adenocarcinoma. Gynecol Oncol Rep. 2014;10:5–8.
49. Misdraji J, Yantiss RK, Graeme-Cook FM, et al. Appendiceal mucinous neoplasms: a clinicopathologic analysis of 107 cases. Am J Surg Pathol. 2003;27:1089–103.
50. Archer AG, Sugarbaker PH, Jelinek JS. Radiology of peritoneal carcinomatosis. In: Sugarbaker PH, editor. Peritoneal carcinomatosis: principles of management. Boston: Kluwer; 1996. p. 263–88.
51. Jacquet P, Jelinek JS, Chang D, et al. Abdominal computed tomographic scan in the selection of patients with mucinous peritoneal carcinomatosis for cytoreductive surgery. J Am Coll Surg. 1995;181:530–8.
52. Yan TD, Haveric N, Carmignani P, Chang D, Sugarbaker PH. Abdominal computed tomography scans in the selection of patients with malignant peritoneal mesothelioma for comprehensive treatment with cytoreductive surgery and perioperative intraperitoneal chemotherapy. Cancer. 2005;15:839–49.
53. Jacquet P, Sugarbaker PH. Current methodologies for clinical assessment of patients with peritoneal carcinomatosis. J Exp Clin Cancer Res. 1996;15:49–58.
54. Sugarbaker PH, Yan TD, Stuart OA, Yoo D. Comprehensive management of diffuse malignant peritoneal mesothelioma. Eur J Surg Oncol. 2006;32:686–91.
55. Deraco M, Nonaka D, Baratti D, et al. Prognostic analysis of clinicopathologic factors in 49 patients with diffuse malignant peritoneal mesothelioma treated with cytoreductive surgery and intraperitoneal hyperthermic perfusion. Ann Surg Oncol. 2006;13:229–37.
56. Elias D, Gilly F, Boutitie F, et al. Peritoneal colorectal carcinomatosis treated with surgery and perioperative intraperitoneal chemotherapy: retrospective analysis of 523 patients from a multicentric French study. J Clin Oncol. 2010;28:63–8.
57. Kalluri R, Weinberg RA. The basics of epithelial-mesenchymal transition. J Clin Invest. 2009;119:1420–8.
58. Sugarbaker PH. Second-look surgery for colorectal cancer: Revised selection factors and new treatment options for greater success. Int J Surg Oncol. 2011; Volume 2011, Article ID 915078, 8 pages, doi:10.1155/2011/915078.
59. Sugarbaker PH. Management of unusual abdominal and pelvic neoplasms with peritoneal dissemination: case reports and literature review. In: Sugarbaker PH, editor. Cytoreductive surgery & perioperative chemotherapy for peritoneal surface malignancy. Textbook and video atlas. Woodbury: Cine-Med Publishing; 2012. p. 137–58.

Chapter 4
Unusual Indications of Cytoreductive Surgery and Hyperthermic Intraperitoneal Chemotherapy: A Review of Outcomes and Report of the Literature

N. Alzahrani, S.J. Valle, W. Liauw, and D.L. Morris

4.1 Introduction

The occurrence of peritoneal carcinomatosis (PC) is serious in all malignancies and usually results in a poor prognosis. Cytoreductive surgery (CRS) and hyperthermic intraperitoneal chemotherapy (HIPEC) is an aggressive surgical approach combining visceral resections and peritonectomy procedures to remove macroscopic disease followed by HIPEC, targeting residual microscopic disease. CRS/HIPEC is the standard and potentially curative treatment for select patients with PC. This combined approach, however, has consistently demonstrated improved survival outcomes across a variety of disease types including appendiceal cancer, colorectal cancer, low-grade appendix mucinous neoplasm, peritoneal mesothelioma and ovarian cancer with peritoneal metastases [1–6], with randomised evidence demonstrating the superiority of CRS/HIPEC for colorectal cancer PC [2]. Although peritonectomy procedures are less likely to achieve disease control in selected patients with significant metastatic disease [7], CRS/HIPEC has been applied and reported in small series of patients with PC of unusual origin including tumours arising from

N. Alzahrani (✉)
Department of Surgery, St George Hospital, Kogarah, NSW 2217, Australia

College of Medicine, Al-Imam Muhammad ibn Saud Islamic University, Riyadh, Saudi Arabia

S.J. Valle • D.L. Morris
Department of Surgery, St George Hospital, Kogarah, NSW 2217, Australia
e-mail: david.morris@unsw.edu.au

W. Liauw
Department of Surgery, St George Hospital, Kogarah, NSW 2217, Australia

Cancer Care Centre, St George Hospital, Kogarah, NSW 2217, Australia

© Springer International Publishing AG 2017
E. Canbay (ed.), *Unusual Cases in Peritoneal Surface Malignancies*,
DOI 10.1007/978-3-319-51523-6_4

sarcoma, desmoplastic small round cell tumour (DSRCT) and neuroendocrine tumours [8–10]. The role of CRS/HIPEC in these patients remains uncertain with limited data on the clinical efficacy of this treatment, as many reports outline specific outcomes in large heterogeneous groups. This goal of this manuscript was to review our single institution experience with CRS/HIPEC for patients with PC of unusual primaries followed by a literature review of studies that reported on greater than five patients of each unusual primary.

4.2 Methods

4.2.1 Patients

From 1,025 patients that underwent CRS/HIPEC at St George Hospital, Australia, between 1996 and 2016, 31 patients had an unusual primary tumour. The tumour included sarcoma ($n = 10$), desmoplastic small round cell tumour ($n = 3$), biliary ($n = 3$), pancreatic ($n = 3$), neuroendocrine ($n = 3$), hepatocellular carcinoma ($n = 3$), primary peritoneal carcinomatosis ($n = 2$), urachal adenocarcinoma ($n = 2$), cystadenoma of the liver ($n = 2$), gastrointestinal stromal tumour ($n = 2$) and breast cancer ($n = 1$). Outcomes were retrospectively reviewed from a prospectively entered database.

4.2.2 Preoperative Management

All patients underwent standard preoperative investigations, which included physical examination; double contrast-enhanced computed tomography (CT) scans of the chest, abdomen and pelvis; and MR study of the liver with Primovist, positron emission tomography and blood tumour markers. All patients were discussed at a multidisciplinary team meeting prior to surgery.

4.3 CRS/HIPEC

An initial assessment of the volume and extent of disease was recorded using the peritoneal carcinomatosis index (PCI), as described by Jacquet and Sugarbaker [11]. CRS was performed using Sugarbaker's technique [11]. All sites and volumes of residual disease following CRS were recorded prospectively using the completeness of cytoreductive (CC) score as previously described [12]. After CRS, HIPEC was performed by installation of a heated chemoperfusate into the abdomen using the coliseum technique at approximately 42 °C, depending on tumour types. However, there is no fixed protocol for PC from unusual primary and was at the discretion of the medical oncologist. Drug choices included cisplatin, mitomycin C and oxaliplatin.

4.3.1   Postoperative Management

Perioperative complications in all patients were graded as previously described [13]. Major morbidity is defined as CDC grade III or IV. All of patients with the aggressive tumour were then followed up at 3-month intervals for the first 12 months and 6-month intervals thereafter until the last time of contact or death. The follow-up review included clinical examination, measurement of relevant tumour markers and assessment of abdominopelvic CT scans.

4.4   Results

The pathology and perioperative outcomes of patients are outlined in Table 4.1. Overall hospital mortality was 5.8% ($n = 2$). Major morbidity rate was 38% ($n = 13$). Mean ICU, HDU and total hospital stay was 4.5 days (standard deviation (SD) = 8.1), 3.0 days (SD = 2.7) and 26.3 days (SD = 21.6), respectively.

Table 4.1 Baseline characteristics of the study cohort

Total n = 34	
Gender n (%)	
Male	18 (52.9)
Female	16 (46.1)
Age mean (SD)	48.4 (14.1)
Primary site	
Cystic adenoma	2 (5.8)
Pancreatic cancer	3 (8.8)
Breast cancer	1 (2.9)
GIST	2 (5.8)
Urachal carcinoma	2 (5.8)
Primary peritoneal cancer	2 (5.8)
Neuroendocrine	3 (8.8)
Biliary adenocarcinoma	3 (5.6)
DSCRT	3 (8.8)
HCC	3 (8.8)
Sarcoma	10 (31.2)
PCI mean (SD)	12.9 (8.3)
CC score	
0	32 (100)
Transfusion mean (SD)	4.4(4.6)
Operation hours mean (SD)	7.4 (2.7)
HIPEC n (%)	
Yes	32 (94.1)
No	2 (5.9)

(continued)

Table 4.1 (continued)

EPIC	
Yes	21 (61.8)
No	13 (38.2)
Mortality rate n (%)	2 (5.8)
Major morbidity rate n (%)	13 (38.2)
ICU stay mean (SD)	4.5 (8.1)
HDU stay mean (SD)	3.0 (2.7)
Total hospital stay mean (SD)	26.3 (21.6)

Table 4.2 Summary of survival (months) for primaries with two or less patients

	Cystic adenoma (n = 2)	Breast cancer (n = 1)	GIST (n = 2)	Urachal carcinoma (n = 2)	Primary peritoneal cancer (n = 2)
Patient 1	0.6 (alive)	0.6 (died)	51.1 (alive)	21.3 (died)	41.4 (died)
Patient 2	12.0 (alive)		4.9 (died)	86.7 (alive)	27.4 (alive)

Table 4.3 Summary of median and overall survival for primaries with at least three patients

	Total number (n)	1-year OS (%)	3-year OS (%)	5-year OS (%)	Median OS (months) (95%CI)	Median DFS (months) (95%CI)
Pancreatic cancer	3	66.7	NR	NR	9.6 (−)	5.2 (−)
Neuroendocrine	3	100.0	33.3	NR	18.9 (0–32.4)	14.6 (−)
Biliary carcinoma	3	33.3	NR	NR	12.0 (−)	3.9 (−)
HCC	3	66.7	33.3	0	36.4 (−)	5.1 (−)
DSRCT	3	100.0	100.0	33.3	64.9 (−)	10.3 (−)
Sarcoma	10	60.0	60.0	0	50.5 (−)	6.6 (1.3–11.9)

NR not reached

Median overall survival (OS) was 29.6 months (95%CI = 13.8–35.5) with a 1-year, 3-year and 5-year survival of 69.6%, 42.7% and 26.7%, respectively. Median follow-up time was 14.4 months (range = 0.2–86.7). Median disease-free survival (DFS) was 6.3 months (95%CI = 2.4–8.1). Survival outcomes by diagnoses and diagnoses with at least three patients were summarised in Tables 4.2 and 4.3, respectively.

4.5 Discussion

4.5.1 Desmoplastic Small Round Cell Tumour

Desmoplastic small round cell tumours (DSRCT) are a rare sarcoma with fewer than 500 cases reported between 1989 and 2015 and is a highly aggressive sarcoma predominantly occurring in males aged between 5 and 35 years [14]. DSRCTs are located almost exclusively in intra-abdominal locations and classically involve a large intra-abdominal mass in the retroperitoneum, pelvis, omentum or mesentery, with diffuse peritoneal deposits that spread along peritoneal and mesothelial surfaces [15, 16]. We previously reported on our patients ($n = 3$) with this tumour and showed a similar outcome [17]. Treatment of isolated peritoneal disease relies on perioperative chemotherapy, most commonly with cisplatin, combined with complete CRS and postoperative radiotherapy [18]. Hayes-Jordan et al. showed that HIPEC has improved survival outcomes with patients receiving neoadjuvant chemotherapy followed by CRS/HIPEC having a 3-year survival of 71% compared to 26% ($p = 0.021$) in patients who did not receive surgery or HIPEC [14]. In a recent study by the same group with the largest experience internationally, the median survival of patients with DSRCT that underwent CRS/HIPEC and complete cytoreduction with no extraabdominal disease was 63.1 months with a 100% 4-year survival [19] (Table 4.4). Our experience of these three patients showed that in concordance with the literature, disease-free survival was 10.3 months although the 3-year survival was 100%. The role of HIPEC for this indication remains controversial; however, complete CRS/HIPEC seems to be an effective therapy for patients with DSCRT.

4.5.2 Peritoneal Sarcomatosis

Approximately 36% of sarcomas originate in the abdominal viscera or retroperitoneum, and metastatic disease is most common to the lungs, liver or directly to peritoneal surfaces and adjacent organs [20]. For patients amenable to resection, local recurrence for abdominal sarcoma ranges from 35% to 82% [21, 22]. Sarcomatosis is defined as the intra-abdominal dissemination of sarcoma and may be present at initial diagnosis but is more frequently observed at recurrence presumably as a result of tumour spillage during the initial resection [23, 24]. When CRS/HIPEC is applied to sarcomatosis, outcomes have been unclear [10, 22, 25–31]. The median overall survival on literature review of peritoneal sarcomatosis post-CRS/HIPEC ranged from 12 to 39.6 months [22, 23, 25–27, 32] (Table 4.4). We report that in our patients, the median overall survival was 50.5 months. Randle et al. [33] reported that although complete cytoreduction is related to improved survival, adding HIPEC in sarcomatosis patients is controversial given the potential toxicity, significant recovery time and lack of a documented benefit. Highly selected sarcomatosis patients are still treated with CRS; however, they are no longer offered HIPEC [33]. A multi-institutional review may be helpful in further defining the role of CRS/HIPEC.

4.6 GIST

Gastrointestinal stromal tumour (GIST) has the highest incidence and prevalence of GI sarcomas, accounting for approximately 5% of all mesenchymal tumours [34]. GISTs may result in sarcomatosis that is chemotherapy resistant, previously leaving patients with few options in the pre-tyrosine kinase inhibitor (TKI) era. The role of

Table 4.4 Literature review of patients with unusual primary that underwent CRS/HIPEC

Author	Year	Primary	Number (n) of patients	Median survival (months)	Disease-free survival (months)	5-year survival
Rossi [22]	2004	Peritoneal sarcomatosis	60	34	22	–
Bonvalot [26]	2005	Peritoneal sarcomatosis	38	29	12.5	45% (1-year survival)
Lim [25]	2007	Peritoneal sarcomatosis	28	5.5–16.9	2.3–4.4	11%
Baratti [9]	2010	Peritoneal sarcomatosis	37	26.2	12.1	24%
Salti [32]	2012	Peritoneal sarcomatosis	13	12	11	–
Randle [33]	2013	Peritoneal sarcomatosis	10	21.6	15.3	43%
Bryan [35]	2015	GIST	18	40	–	56% (3-year survival)
Hayes-Jordan [14]	2010	DSRCT	24	12.4	12	71%
Hayes-Jordan [19]	2014	DSRCT	26	31.1	–	–
Honore [18]	2015	DSRCT	23	25.7	15.5	–
Elias [8]	2014	Neuroendocrine tumour	41	NR	–	69%
Tentes [61]	2012	Pancreatic adenocarcinoma	21	11	5	23%
Bakrin [53]	2013	Primary peritoneal carcinomatosis	36	NR	16.7	57.4%
Tabrizian [58]	2014	Hepatocellular carcinoma	14	35.6 (CC0/1)	23	–
Krane [51]	2012	Urachal carcinoma	5	27	13	–
Cardi [37]	2013	Breast carcinoma	5	63.2	NR	–

NR not reached, *DSCRT* desmoplastic small round cell tumour, *GIST* gastrointestinal stromal tumour

– not recorded

patients received different intraperitoneal chemotherapy regimens surgery for metastatic GIST in the post-TKI era remains uncertain. Bryan et al. [35] reported a median survival in patients who progressed on a TKI preoperatively was 1.35 years post-CRS/HIPEC as compared with a median survival that was not reached in those without progression on TKIs ($p = 0.007$). The median overall survival for the entire cohort was 3.33 years post-CRS/HIPEC (Table 4.4). Of our two patients, one died at 4.9 months post-CRS/HIPEC and one was alive and well at 51.1 months. Studies indicate that CRS in those who have progressed on preoperative TKIs yields a poor outcome with a median survival of 1.09 years, which was evident in our short-surviving patient. It is suggested that offering CRS in patients with GIST sarcomatosis who on preoperative imaging have disease response or are stable on TKIs may be considered and should be performed in highly selected patients before developing TKI resistance [35, 36]. Progression on a TKI seems to be associated with poor outcomes even after a complete cytoreduction [36].

4.6.1   Breast Cancer

PC from breast cancer is rare [37–39], and no clear guidelines are available regarding the role of CRS ± HIPEC for these patients [40, 41]. A median of 18 years (range 10–30) elapsed after breast cancer was diagnosed and PC developed. Previous reports describe breast cancer as one of the most slowly growing solid tumours given that metastases may appear even decades after the initial diagnosis [41, 42]. In one CRS study, of the five patients treated, four achieved long-term survival, one surviving even for 10 years with good quality of life [37, 42] (Table 4.2). Our single breast cancer patient died on day 18 postoperatively from sepsis. No clear guidelines are reported in literature regarding the treatment of these patients because cases are sporadic and rarely referred. Cisplatin is one of the most common chemotherapy agents used for HIPEC [43]. The long disease-free and overall survival observed in our small series suggests that in highly selected patients with no extraperitoneal disease and in whom surgery can achieve adequate cytoreduction this combined procedure is a promising approach for patients with PC from breast cancer.

4.6.2   Mucinous Carcinoma of the Urachus

The urachus is a remnant of foetal development that can give rise to benign or malignant mucinous tumours [44]. Extension of these tumours into the peritoneal cavity results in a clinical picture similar to pseudomyxoma peritonei (PMP). Most urachal tumours are adenocarcinoma, and approximately 70% of urachal carcinomas are mucin producing [45]. With disease progression, mucin accumulates, leaks from the tumour and ruptured urachus and spreads through the peritoneal cavity. A 5-year survival rate has been reported in up to 40% of patients [46–48]. The standard approach for urachal tumours is to treat like PMP, by complete CRS/HIPEC, which has been reported to significantly improve patients' survival and prognosis [3, 49, 50, 51]. In 28 reported cases, 15 patients undergoing CRS/HIPEC had a median disease-free survival of 25 months. Honore et al. [44] reported on three patients; two were alive and disease-free at 20 and 37 months. The third patient developed early peritoneal recurrence and died after 14 months. All five patients reported by Krane et al. [51] successfully completed CRS/HIPEC with mitomycin C but developed local or distant disease recurrence at a median of 13 months postoperatively (range 7–31) and median survival of 27 months (range 21–87) (Table 4.4). Our survival and recurrence data on the two patients are similar to these studies. As a result, we suggest that CRS/HIPEC can be considered in selected patients as a new option of treatment for PMP from urachus.

4.6.3   Primary Peritoneal Tumour

Primary peritoneal serous carcinoma is a very rare form of PC, occurring almost exclusively in females; however, the incidence is unknown [44, 52]. The largest study described 36 patients from nine European centres. After complete CRS/ HIPEC, it reported an overall 1-, 3- and 5-year survival of 94%, 72% and 57%, respectively, with a median recurrence-free survival of 17 months [53] (Table 4.4). There is no comparative study to determine whether CRS/HIPEC is of benefit to patients with primary peritoneal carcinoma. Both of our patients showed similar outcomes and these in comparison to reported survival and recurrence to those with epithelioid mesothelioma from our centre are similar [54], therefore we can suggest, along with others [53], that CRS/HIPEC be considered in patients with this tumour.

4.6.4   Hepatocellular Carcinoma

Hepatocellular carcinoma (HCC) represents the major subtype accounting for up to 85% of primary liver cancers [55]. A subgroup of patients with HCC presents with peritoneal metastasis; the incidence of this is approximately 18% based on autopsy findings [56, 57]. The largest study reported by Lin et al. [10] investigated the survival of 53 HCC patients with peritoneal disease. The majority presented as a metachronous peritoneal recurrence (81.1%). CRS was offered to a select group of patients (65.1%) either with or without combined repeat hepatectomy. Median survival of patients undergoing CRS was 12.5 months compared to 2.1 months with systemic chemotherapy alone. Tabrizian et al. [58] reported following CRS/HIPEC that the time to metachronous peritoneal recurrence was 23 months. The 3-year recurrence rate was 100%, and the median survival of the cohort that had a complete cytoreduction was 35.6 months (Table 4.4). CRS/HIPEC appears superior compared to systemic chemotherapy alone in the treatment of peritoneal dissemination of HCC. Our experience also shows comparable results, and, although all our patients recurred within 6 months, we report a median survival of 36.4 months. PC reflects locoregional spread rather than systemic dissemination; it would therefore be warranted to further investigate the role of HIPEC in the treatment of peritoneal HCC.

4.6.5 Pancreatic Adenocarcinoma

Unfortunately, only 10–20% of patients diagnosed with pancreatic cancer are able to undergo potentially curative surgery [59]. Furthermore, long-term 5- or 10-year survival is rare, even after potentially curative complete resection, where disease recurrence has been documented in the local and regional area (50%), on peritoneal surfaces (40–60%) and within the liver as hepatic metastases (50–60%) [60]. The results of adjuvant treatment either with chemotherapy or with radiotherapy have been contradictory, and the incidence of local-regional recurrence remains high [61]. It has been shown both from laboratory and clinical studies that the intraperitoneal use of gemcitabine may effectively target local disease not only locoregionally but also in the portal venous circulation [62]. Tentes et al. [61] reported on 21 patients that underwent CRS/HIPEC with gemcitabine. The 5-year and median survival was 23% and 11 months, respectively. The recurrence rate was 50%, but no patient developed local-regional recurrence, which is quite remarkable. We report a median survival of 9.6 months. These limited results do suggest that patients with pancreatic cancer undergoing potentially curative resection in combination with gemcitabine HIPEC may be offered a survival benefit, and data suggested that local-regional recurrences may be greatly reduced by the application of HIPEC [61, 63].

4.6.6 Neuroendocrine Carcinomas

Neuroendocrine tumours (NET) are well-differentiated, hormonally active tumours. NET-derived peritoneal carcinomatosis arises mainly from gastrointestinal tumours and usually represents only a small part of the tumour load. NETs are associated with other sites of distant metastases, notably liver metastases. In addition, in 60–70% of patients, the resection or ablation of multiple liver metastases is required. The incidence of PC from NET is approximately 17% [64, 65]. Our limited data shows that all three of our patients were alive at 1 year; however, one died shortly after from an unrelated illness. Elias et al. [8] reported in 50 patients that underwent complete resection with CRS ± HIPEC and showed an overall survival at 5 and 10 years of 69% and 52%, respectively, and disease-free survival at 5 and 10 years of 17% and 6%, respectively. At 5 years, PC and liver metastases recurred in 47% and in 66% of cases, respectively. Overall survival was not significant between patients treated with or without HIPEC; however, disease-free survival was greater in the

HIPEC group (p = 0.018), which was attributed to lower systemic disease (Table 4.4). Despite limitations of this study and limited literature available, these results suggest that CRS may be feasible. The benefit of HIPEC in addition to CRS is, however, unclear. HIPEC offers the theoretic advantage of eradicating residual disease after CRS, although Elias reported no observed difference between the HIPEC and non-HIPEC group in terms of survival, the incidence of liver recurrences and the incidence of peritoneal recurrences [66]. The use of HIPEC should therefore be at the discretion of the multidisciplinary team.

4.6.7   Biliary Carcinomas

Gallbladder cancer is the most common malignant tumour of the biliary tract worldwide [66]. It is also the most aggressive cancer of the biliary tract with the shortest median survival from the time of diagnosis [67]. This poor prognosis is due, in part, to an aggressive biologic behaviour and a lack of sensitive screening tests for early detection resulting in delayed diagnosis at advanced stage [68]. Intraperitoneal spread is common with ascites, omental nodules and peritoneal implants occurring in 24.6% of cases [66, 69, 70]. Surgical resection may provide cure; however, at initial presentation, only 10% of patients are candidates for surgery with a curative intent [67, 71]. Our patients had a poor disease-free survival of 3.9 months although did have a median survival of 12 months. A randomised trial compared systemic chemotherapy of gemcitabine plus oxaliplatin or 5-FU plus leucovorin versus best supportive care alone in 81 patients with unresectable gallbladder cancer and showed the median overall survival in best supportive care and 5-FU/leucovorin groups was 4.5 and 4.6 months, respectively, versus 9.5 months in gemcitabine plus oxaliplatin group [72]. A pooled analysis of 104 chemotherapy trials involving 1,368 patients with biliary tract and gallbladder cancers showed superior response rate for gallbladder cancer compared with cholangiocarcinoma (36 versus 18%) but shorter overall survival for gallbladder cancer (7.2 versus 9.3 months) [73]. Patients with gallbladder cancer and cholangiocarcinoma with PC are not yet established as good candidates for CRS/HIPEC due to the very limited number of patients reported in literature as results tend to be reported as a heterogeneous cohort. Further studies are required to establish the potential benefit of CRS/HIPEC.

4.7   Conclusion

The finding of peritoneal dissemination from unusual primaries should not be a contraindication for CRS/HIPEC. The selection of patients suitable for this treatment option is difficult. It is also difficult to draw conclusion on survival benefits provided by CRS/HIPEC due to the small number of patients in each group. Due to the rarity of these conditions, a randomised controlled trial comparing CRS/HIPEC is not plausible. A larger cohort is necessary to become aware of outcomes following CRS/HIPEC. A multicentre review of each unusual primary is warranted to establish the benefit, or otherwise, of CRS ± HIPEC.

References

1. Yan TD, Deraco M, Baratti D, et al. Cytoreductive surgery and hyperthermic intraperitoneal chemotherapy for malignant peritoneal mesothelioma: a multi-institutional experience. J Clin Oncol. 2009;27:6237–42.
2. Verwaal VJ, van Ruth S, de Bree E, et al. Randomized trial of cytoreduction and hyperthermic intraperitoneal chemotherapy versus systemic chemotherapy and palliative surgery in patients with peritoneal carcinomatosis of colorectal cancer. J Clin Oncol. 2003;21:3737–42.
3. Chua TC, Moran BJ, Sugarbaker PH, et al. Early- and long-term outcome data of patients with pseudomyxoma peritonei from appendiceal origin treated by a strategy of cytoreductive surgery and hyperthermic intraperitoneal chemotherapy. J Clin Oncol. 2012;30:2449–56.
4. Glehen O, Gilly FN, Boutitie F, et al. Toward curative treatment of peritoneal carcinomatosis from nonovarian origin by cytoreductive surgery combined with perioperative intraperitoneal chemotherapy: a multi-institutional study of 1290 patients. Cancer. 2010;116:5608–18.
5. Deraco M, Baratti D, Laterza B, et al. Advanced cytoreduction as surgical standard of care and hyperthermic intraperitoneal chemotherapy as promising treatment in epithelial ovarian cancer. Eur J Surg Oncol. 2011;37:4–9.
6. Elias D, Glehen O, Pocard M, et al. A comparative study of complete cytoreductive surgery plus intraperitoneal chemotherapy to treat peritoneal dissemination from colon, rectum, small bowel and non pseudomyxoma appendix. Ann Surg. 2010;251:896–901.
7. Sugarbaker PH. Intraperitoneal chemotherapy and cytoreductive surgery for the prevention and treatment of peritoneal carcinomatosis and sarcomatosis. Semin Surg Oncol. 1998;14:254–61.
8. Elias D, David A, Sourrouille I, Honoré C, Goéré D, Dumon F, et al. Neuroendocrine carcinomas: optimal surgery of peritoneal metastasis (and associated intra-abdominal metastasis). Surgery. 2014;15(1):5–12.
9. Baratti D, Pennacchioli E, Kusamura S, Fiore M, Balestra MR, Colombo C, et al. Peritoneal sarcomatosis: is there a subset of patients who may benefit from cytoreductive surgery and hyperthermic intraperitoneal chemotherapy? Ann Surg Oncol. 2012;17:3220–8.
10. Kalliampust AA, Shukla NK, Deo SV, Yadav P, Mudaly D, Yadav R, et al. Updates on the multimodality management of desmoplastic small round cell tumors. J Surg Oncol. 2012;105:617–21.
11. Sugarbaker PH. Peritonectomy procedures. Ann Surg. 1995;221(1):29–42.
12. Jacquet P, Sugarbaker PH. Clinical research methodologies in diagnosis and staging of patients with peritoneal carcinomatosis. Peritoneal carcinomatosis: principles of management. Springer; United States of America. 1996. p. 359–74.
13. Dindo D, Demartines N, Clavien P-A. Classification of surgical complications: a new proposal with evaluation in a cohort of 6336 patients and results of a survey. Ann Surg. 2004; 240(2):205.
14. Hayes-Jordan A, Green H, Fitzgerald N, Xiao L, Anderson P. Novel treatment for desmoplastic small round cell tumor: hyperthermic intraperitoneal perfusion. J Pediatr Surg. 2010;45(5):1000–6.
15. Hayes-Jordan A, Pappo A. Management of desmoplastic small round-cell tumors in children and young adults. J Pediatr Hematol Oncol. 2012;34(Suppl. 2):S73–5.
16. Gerald WL, Miller HK, Battifora H, Miettinen M, Silva EG, Rosai J. Intra-abdominal desmoplastic small round-cell tumor. Report of 19 cases of a distinctive type of high-grade polyphenotypic malignancy affecting young individuals. Am J Surg Pathol. 1991;15(6):499–513.

17. Fan H, I'Ons B, McConnell R, et al. Peritonectomy and hyperthermic intraperitoneal chemotherapy as treatment for desmoplastic small round cell tumour. Int J Surg Case Rep. 2015;7:85–8.
18. Honore C, Amroun K, Vilcot L, et al. Abdominal desmoplastic small round cell tumour: multimodal treatment combining chemotherapy, surgery and radiotherapy is the best option. Ann Surg Oncol. 2015;22:1073–9.
19. Hayes-Jordan A, Green HL, Lin H, et al. Complete cytoreduction and HIPEC improves survival in desmoplastic small round cell tumor. Ann Surg Oncol. 2014;21:220–4.
20. Singer S, Maki RG, O'Sullivan B. Soft tissue sarcoma. In: De Vita Jr VT, Lawrence TS, Rosenberg SA, et al., editors. Cancer: principles & practice of oncology. Philadelphia: Wolters Kluwer Health/Lippincott Williams & Wilkins; 2011. p. 1533–77.
21. Mudan SS, Conlon KC, Woodruff JM, et al. Salvage surgery for patients with recurrent gastrointestinal sarcoma: prognostic factors to guide patient selection. Cancer. 2000;88: 66–74.
22. Rossi CR, Deraco M, De SM, et al. Hyperthermic intraperitoneal intraoperative chemotherapy after cytoreductive surgery for the treatment of abdominal sarcomatosis: clinical outcome and prognostic factors in 60 consecutive patients. Cancer. 2004;100:1943–50.
23. Karakousis CP, Blumenson LE, Canavese G, et al. Surgery for disseminated abdominal sarcoma. Am J Surg. 1992;163:560–4.
24. Bilimoria MM, Holtz DJ, Mirza NQ, et al. Tumor volume as a prognostic factor for sarcomatosis. Cancer. 2002;94:2441–6.
25. Lim SJ, Cormier JN, Feig BW, et al. Toxicity and outcomes associated with surgical cytoreduction and hyperthermic intraperitoneal chemotherapy (HIPEC) for patients with sarcomatosis. Ann Surg Oncol. 2007;14:2309–18.
26. Bonvalot S, Cavalcanti A, Le PC, et al. Randomized trial of cytoreduction followed by intraperitoneal chemotherapy versus cytoreduction alone in patients with peritoneal sarcomatosis. Eur J Surg Oncol. 2005;31:917–23.
27. Seo CJ, Tan GHC, Soo KC, Teo MC. Cytoreductive sugery and hyperthermic intraperitoneal chemotherapy: unconventional indications. EC Cancer. 2015:25–7.
28. Huh WW, Fitzgerald NE, Mahajan A, et al. Peritoneal sarcomatosis in pediatric malignancies. Pediatr Blood Cancer. 2013;60:12–7.
29. Munene G, Mack LA, Temple WJ. Systematic review on the efficacy of multimodal treatment of sarcomatosis with cytoreduction and intraperitoneal chemotherapy. Ann Surg Oncol. 2011;18:207–13.
30. Rossi CR, Casali P, Kusamura S, et al. The consensus statement on the locoregional treatment of abdominal sarcomatosis. J Surg Oncol. 2008;98:291–4.
31. Sugarbaker PH. Review of a personal experience in the management of carcinomatosis and sarcomatosis. Jpn J Clin Oncol. 2001;31:573–83.
32. Salti GI, Ailabouni L, Undevia S. Cytoreductive surgery and hyperthermic intraperitoneal chemotherapy for the treatment of peritoneal sarcomatosis. Ann Surg Oncol. 2012;19:1410–5.
33. Randle RW, Swett KR, Shen P, et al. Cytoreductive surgery with hyperthermic intraperitoneal chemotherapy in peritoneal sarcomatosis. Am Surg. 2014;79(6):620–4.
34. Perez EA, Livingstone AS, Franceschi D, et al. Current incidence and outcomes of gastrointestinal mesenchymal tumors including gastrointestinal stromal tumors. J Am Coll Surg. 2006;202:623–9.
35. Bryan ML, Fitzgerald NC, Levine EA, et al. Cytoreductive surgery with hyperthermic intraperitoneal chemotherapy in sarcomatosis from gastrointestinal stromal tumour. Am Surg. 2014;80(9):890–5.
36. Turley RS, Peng PD, Reddy SK, et al. Hepatic resection for metastatic gastrointestinal stromal tumours in the tyrosine kinase inhibitor era. Cancer. 2011;118:3571–8.
37. Cardi M, Sammartino P, Framarino ML, Biacchi D, Cortesi E, Sibio S, et al. Treatment of peritoneal carcinomatosis from breast cancer by maximal cytoreduction and HIPEC: a preliminary report on 5 cases. Breast. 2013;22:845–9.

38. Tuthill M, Pell R, Giuliani R, Lim A, Gudi M, Contractor KB, et al. Peritoneal disease in breast cancer: a specific entity with an extremely poor prognosis. Eur J Cancer. 2009;45:2146–9.
39. Stebbing J, Crane J, Gaya A. Breast cancer (metastatic). Clin Evid. 2006;15:2331–59.
40. Eitan R, Gemignani ML, Verkatraman ES, Barakat RR, Abu-Rustrum NR, et al. Breast cancer metastatic to abdomen and pelvis. Role of surgical resection. Gynecol Oncol. 2003;90:397–401.
41. Abu-Rustum NR, Aghajanian CA, Venkatraman ES, Feroz F, Barakat RR. Metastatic breast carcinoma to the abdomen and pelvis. Gynecol Oncol. 1997;66:41–4.
42. Sheen-Chen SM, Liu YW, Sun CK, Lin SE, Eng HI, Huang WT, et al. Abdominal carcinomatosis attributed to metastatic breast carcinoma. Dig Dis Sci. 2008;53:3043–5.
43. Cardi M, Sammartino P, Mingarelli V, et al. Cytoreduction and HIPEC in the treatment of "unconventional" secondary peritoneal carcinomatosis. World J Surg Oncol. 2015;13:305.
44. Honore C, Goere D, Macovei R, Colace L, Benhaim L, Elias D. Peritoneal carcinomatosis from unusual cancer origins: is there a role for hyperthermic intraperitoneal chemotherapy? J Visc Surg. 2016;153:101–7.
45. Sheldon CA, Clayman RV, Gonzalez R, Williams RD, Fraley EE. Malignant urachal lesions. J Urol. 1984;131:1–8.
46. Ashley RA, Inman BA, Sebo TJ, Leibovich BC, Blute ML, Kwon ED, Zincke H. Urachal carcinoma: clinicopathologic features and long-term outcomes of an aggressive malignancy. Cancer. 2006;107:712–20.
47. Henly DR, Farrow GM, Zincke H. Urachal cancer: role of conservative surgery. Urology. 1993;42:635–9.
48. Siefker-Radtke AO, Gee J, Shen Y, Wen S, Daliani D, Millikan RE, Pisters LL. Multimodality management of urachal carcinoma: the MD Anderson Cancer Center experience. J Urol. 2003;169:1295–8.
49. Sugarbaker PH, Jablonski KA. Prognostic features of 51 colorectal and 130 appendiceal cancer patients with peritoneal carcinomatosis treated by cytoreductive surgery and intraperitoneal chemotherapy. Ann Surg. 1995;221:124–32.
50. Miner TJ, Shia J, Jaques DP, Klimstra DS, Brennan MF, Coit DG. Long-term survival following treatment of pseudomyxoma peritonei: an analysis of surgical therapy. Ann Surg. 2005;241:300–8.
51. Krane LS, Kader AK, Levine EA. Cytoreductive surgery with hyperthermic intraperitoneal chemotherapy for patients with peritoneal carcinomatosis secondary to urachal adenocarcinoma. J Surg Oncol. 2012;105(3):258–60.
52. Swerdlow M. Mesothelioma of the pelvic peritoneum resembling papillary cystadenocarcinoma of the ovary. Am J Obstet Gynecol. 1959;77:197–200.
53. Bakrin N, Gilly FN, Baratti D, et al. Primary peritoneal serous carcinoma treated by cytoreductive surgery combined with hyperthermic intraperitoneal chemotherapy. A multi-institutional study of 36 patients. Eur J Surg Oncol. 2013;39:742–7.
54. Huang Y, Alzahrani N, Liauw W, Morris DL. Repeat cytoreductive surgery and hyperthermic intraperitoneal chemotherapy for recurrent diffuse malignant peritoneal mesothelioma. Eur J Surg Oncol. 2015;41(10):1373–8.
55. Jemal A, Bray F, Center MM, et al. Global cancer statistics. Cancer J Clin. 2011;61:69–90.
56. Chua TC, Morris DL. Exploring the role of resection of extrahepatic metastases from hepatocellular carcinoma. Surg Oncol. 2012;21:95–101.
57. Lin CC, Liang HP, Lee HS, et al. Clinical manifestations and survival of hepatocellular carcinoma patients with peritoneal metastasis. J Gastroenterol Hepatol. 2009;24:815–20.
58. Tabrizian P, Franssen B, Jibara G, et al. Cytoreductive surgery with or without hyperthermic intraperitoneal chemotherapy in patients with peritoneal hepatocellular carcinoma. J Surg Oncol. 2014;110:786–90.
59. Schneider G, Siveke JT, Eckel F, Schmid RM. Pancreatic cancer: basic and clinical aspects. Gastroenterology. 2005;128(6):1606–25.
60. Warshaw AL, Fernandez-Del CC. Medical progress: pancreatic carcinoma. N Engl J Med. 1992;326(7):455–65.

61. Tentes AAK, Kyzirdis D, Kakolyris S, et al. Preliminary results of hyperthermic intraperitoneal intraoperative chemotherapy as an adjuvant in resectable pancreatic cancer. Gastroenterol Res Pract. 2012;2012:506571.
62. Ridwelski K, Meyer F, Hribaschek A, Kasper U, Lippert H. Intraoperative and early postoperative chemotherapy into the abdominal cavity using gemcitabine may prevent postoperative occurrence of peritoneal carcinomatosis. J Surg Oncol. 2002;79(1):10–6.
63. Sugarbaker PH, Stuart AO, Bijelic L. Intraperitoneal gemcitabine chemotherapy treatment for patients with resected pancreatic cancer: rationale and report on early data. Int J Surg Oncol. 2011;2-11:161862.
64. Mitry E, O'Toole D, Louvet C, et al. Resultats de l'enquete nationale FFCD-ANGH-GERCOR sur les tumerus endocrines a localization digestive. Gastroenterol Clin Biol. 2003;27:A135.
65. Norlen O, Stalberg P, Oberg K, et al. Long-term results of surgery for small intestinal neuroendocrine tumors in a tertiary referral centre. Would J Surg. 2012;36:1419–31.
66. Lai CHE, Lau WY. Gallbladder cancer—a comprehensive review. Surgeon. 2008;6(2):101–10. doi:10.1016/s1479-666x(08)80073-x.
67. Zhu AX, Hong TS, Hezel AF, Kooby DA. Current management of gallbladder carcinoma. Oncologist. 2010;15(2):168–81. doi:10.1634/theoncologist.2009-0302.
68. Dutta U. Gallbladder cancer: can newer insights improve the outcome? J Gastroenterol Hepatol. 2012;27(4):642–53. doi:10.1111/j.1440-1746.2011.07048.x.
69. Wu K, Liao M, Liu B, Deng Z. ADAM-17 over-expression in gallbladder carcinoma correlates with poor prognosis of patients. Med Oncol. 2011;28(2):475–80.
70. Andrén-Sandberg Å. Molecular biology of gallbladder cancer: potential clinical implications. N Am J Med Sci. 2012;4(10):435–41.
71. Spiliotis J, Halika E, de Bree E. Treatment of peritoneal surface malignancies with hyperthermic intraperitoneal chemotherapy – current perspectives. Curr Oncol. 2016;23(3):e266–75.
72. Sharma A, Dwary AD, Mohanti BK, et al. Best supportive care compared with chemotherapy for unresectable gall bladder cancer: a randomized controlled study. J Clin Oncol. 2010;28(30):4581–6.
73. Eckel F, Schmid RM. Chemotherapy in advanced biliary tract carcinoma: a pooled analysis of clinical trials. Br J Cancer. 2007;96(6):896–902.

Chapter 5
Management of Desmoplastic Small Round Cell Tumor

Andrea Hayes-Jordan

5.1 Introduction

DSRCT is a very newly described tumor, characterized in 1989 by Gerald and Rosai, who identified the EWS-WT1 translocation and fusion protein as pathognomonic. If this fusion protein cannot be identified in the tissue, the diagnosis of DSRCT cannot be made. DSRCT was a relatively unknown tumor that was considered by most clinicians to be an aggressive rare sarcoma that was lethal. Identifying the pathology and characteristic translocation was of key importance to developing any treatment strategies [1, 2]. Gerald and Rosai described not only the characteristic translocation but also the histologic appearance. Nests of small round blue cells can be seen separated by desmoplastic stroma (Fig. 5.1). The translocation (11:22), (p13:q12) and the fusion protein of Ewing's sarcoma (EWS) and Wilms' tumor (WT-1), makes the diagnosis [1–3]. Confirming this translocation to make the diagnosis of DSRCT, by percutaneous or open biopsy, is necessary. The five survivals are estimated only at 15–30% [1–3]. If the EWS translocation is not identified, the diagnosis becomes challenging. One author describes the desmin reactivity and cytokeratin staining can be seen in either blastemal predominant Wilms' tumor or DSRCT. Detection of an EWSR1-WT1 rearrangement and selective WT1 carboxy-terminus immunoreactivity (characteristic of DSRCT) or dual immunoreactivity for the WT1 amino-terminus and carboxy-terminus (characteristic of WT) remain the most discriminating diagnostic tools [4].

A. Hayes-Jordan, MD
The University of Texas MD Anderson Cancer Center, Department of Surgical Oncology,
1400 Pressler St., Unit 1484, Houston, TX 77030, USA
e-mail: ahjordan@mdanderson.org

© Springer International Publishing AG 2017
E. Canbay (ed.), *Unusual Cases in Peritoneal Surface Malignancies*,
DOI 10.1007/978-3-319-51523-6_5

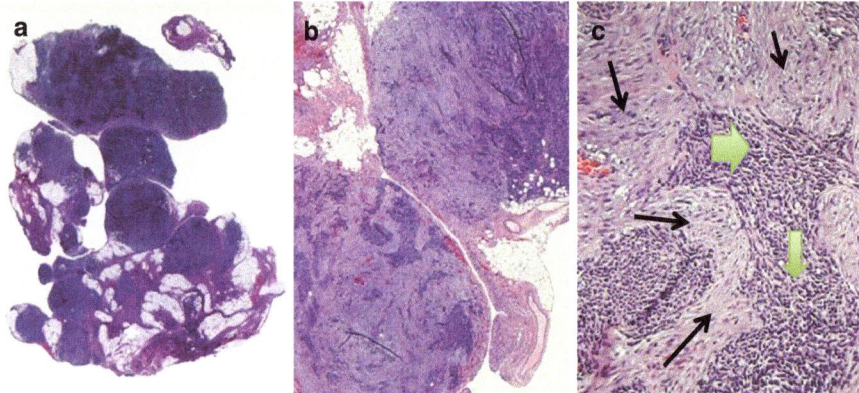

Fig. 5.1 Low- (**a**-5 and **b**-20×) and high-power (**c**-40×) histologic sections of DSRCT from an omental biopsy. In figure (**c**), nests of small round blue cells (*filled arrow*) interdigitate between bands of fibrous stroma (*line arrow*)

5.2 Diagnosis and Staging

The age of presentation is typically 5–30 years, and 85–90% of the patients are male [5].

Large masses, in addition to visceral and parietal seeding of the peritoneum, are a typical presentation in DSRCT. Usually vague abdominal pain brings this to the attention of the patient and prompts imaging examinations. The dissemination of DSRCT throughout the abdominal cavity is characteristic. The reason a large tumor burden exists at diagnosis is few symptoms are present until the peritoneal surfaces are infiltrated with tumor and overwhelm the peritoneum, therefore impairing resorption of peritoneal fluid and causing ascites. Abdominal distension and discomfort are the usual presenting symptoms. Patients can also have pain and constipation. Because of the sarcomatosis seen, these patients are considered Stage 4 at diagnosis. It is rare for a patient to present with a single mass or one or two masses. This only occurs when the mass is found incidentally at the time of another operation or diagnostic radiologic exam for another entity.

Because of the frequent diffuse nature of the presentation of this disease, a new staging system is being considered, and now being used on a trial basis, by Hayes-Jordan and colleagues at MD Anderson Cancer Center. In this proposed staging system, Stage 1 patients would have limited disease, localized to one or two sites in the abdomen or one site elsewhere. Stage 2 patients would have any amount of extensive peritoneal disease; Stage 3, with liver metastasis and peritoneal disease; and Stage 4 with peritoneal and liver disease and disease also outside of the abdominal cavity, including lymph nodes. This has not been validated and is under investigation.

5.3 Imaging Characteristics

On initial imaging, typically, CT (computed tomography) scans are done. MRI and ultrasound can also be helpful. On CT scan or MRI, usually multiple peritoneal implants can be seen, making the diagnosis of DSRCT highly suspicious. The most common site of initial organ metastasis is usually the liver. The lungs, pleura, and mediastinum are the next most common locations for metastasis. Lymph node enlargement in the groin and neck can also be seen. Therefore, PET (positron-emission tomography) scan imaging may be a helpful adjunct to evaluate distant metastasis at the time of staging [6].

The extent of disease seen on initial imaging includes many lesions in every portion of the peritoneal cavity. The most common areas are the omentum, right diaphragm, and pelvis (Fig. 5.2). The splenic hilum and various small bowel and colon mesenteric implants are also common. Retroperitoneal disease is very uncommon. In most cases, the disease seen on CT or MRI imaging underestimates the extent of the diseases. One to 2 mm metastasis and "sheets" of tumor in confluence are common intraoperative findings (Fig. 5.3). Metastatic disease outside of the abdominal cavity can be found in the mediastinum, pleura, supradiaphragmatic lymph nodes, lung, and bone.

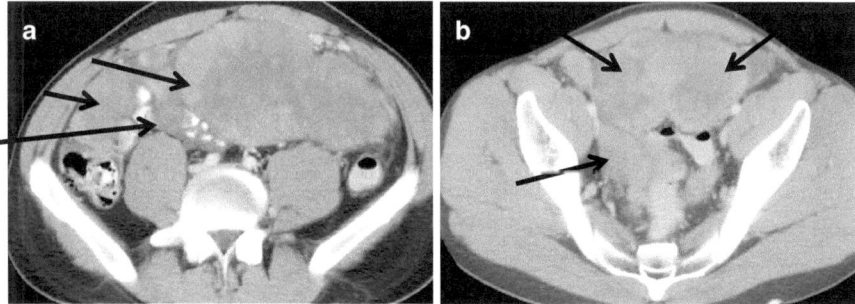

Fig. 5.2 Figure (**a**) shows a large omental mass in a newly diagnosed patient with DSRCT. Figure (**b**) shows a pelvic, paravesical mass, large and lobulated. Pelvic tumors are very typical of DSRCT sarcomatosis

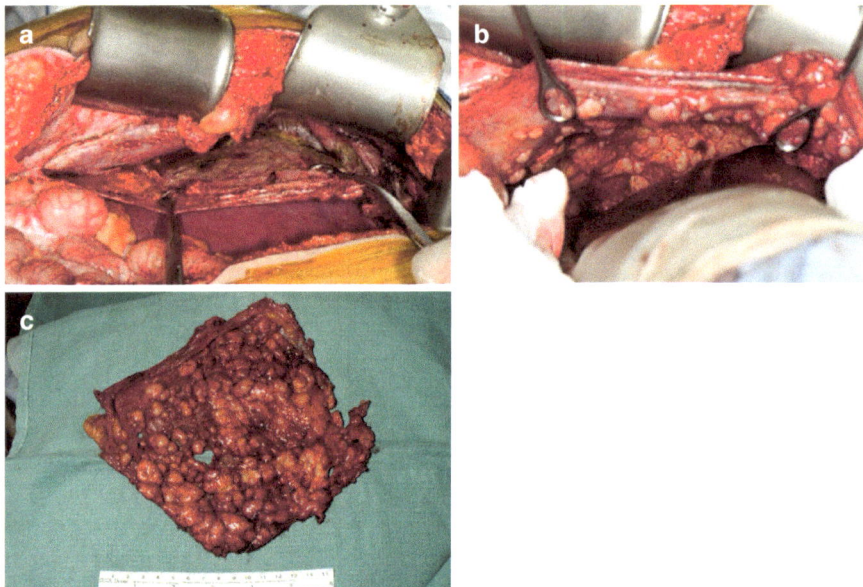

Fig. 5.3 A "sheet" of sarcomatosis from DSRCT in the right diaphragm peritoneum. Figure (**a, b**) show the intraoperative dissection of the right diaphragm peritoneum. The final result (**c**) is one "sheet" of tumor without any diaphragm muscle removed

5.4   Chemotherapy

Since its description in 1989 by Gerald and Rosai at Memorial Sloan Kettering Cancer Center, multimodality chemotherapy has been used for DSRCT. Ewing's type chemotherapy, aggressive surgery, tumor debulking, total abdominal radiation therapy, and high-dose chemotherapy followed by autologous stem cell rescue have all been used in the treatment of DSRCT, with little improvement in survival. Durable remissions remain rare [7]. Control of DSRCT with chemotherapy is most effective in children, with Ewing's type chemotherapy. Ewing's type chemotherapy is the standard because efficacy with this regimen has been demonstrated by Kushner et al. [7]. This chemotherapy is based on alkylating agents cyclophosphamide or ifosfamide along with vincristine and doxorubicin alternating with ifosfamide and etoposide. This regimen was shown to have a favorable outcome in a multidisciplinary approach in 12 DSRCT patients [7]. This chemotherapy regimen was used in combination with aggressive surgical complete excision and postoperative whole abdominal radiation, providing improved survival. With a median follow-up of 22 months, the median disease-free survival was 19 months. The regimen can be quite toxic, and frequent admissions for fever and myelosuppression can be expected. An alternative more tolerable outpatient regimen has been utilized [8]. This includes neoadjuvant vincristine, ifosfamide, dexrazoxane/doxorubicin, and etoposide. This is followed be aggressive surgical excision and removal of all gross disease, including 1–2 mm peritoneal implants. This was followed by adjuvant radiotherapy (30 Gy whole abdomen) and irinotecan and Temodar for a total of 12 cycles. This regimen yielded a disease-free interval of approximately 2 years. The irinotecan and Temodar therapy provided an excellent quality of life with regular school attendance and participation in plan activities. This regimen may be used after surgery and radiotherapy [8].

5.5 Surgical Therapy

As mentioned, abdominal sarcomatosis is a common finding with tumor implants ranging from 1 mm to 40 cm or more. The extent of disease seen on initial imaging includes many lesions in every portion of the peritoneal cavity. Typically, omental disease is found in most patients in addition to peritoneal studding on the diaphragm, spleen, Morison's pouch, abdominal wall peritoneum, small bowel mesentery, and almost certainly in the pelvis. Peritonectomies are required in these locations for effective complete gross resection and cytoreduction. In most cases, the disease seen on CT or MRI imaging underestimates the extent of the diseases. One to 2 mm metastasis and "sheets" of tumor in confluence are common intraoperative findings.

Because this is usually a very chemo-responsive tumor, the feasibility of surgical resection should not be assessed until a plateau of response from chemotherapy has been reached. This is usually achieved after 4–6 months of neoadjuvant chemotherapy. The partial response to neoadjuvant chemotherapy in DSRCT is an important component to complete surgical resection. In a report of the impact of complete surgical resection of DSRCT, LaQuaglia and colleagues found a 3-year overall survival of 58% with complete resection and 0% when resection was not done, and the patients were treated with chemotherapy and radiotherapy alone [5].

In this setting, even after surgical resection of gross, visible disease, and cytoreduction, microscopic residual can be expected. Hence, a regional approach to local control such as hyperthermic intraperitoneal chemotherapy (HIPEC) could be an effective strategy for DSRCT. HIPEC is a potential adjunct to complete surgical resection of DSRCT. Figure 5.4. shows a schemata of a typical HIPEC setup, including the infusion of heated chemotherapy (41.5 °C) which occurs over a 90-min period in the operating room after complete cytoreduction (Fig. 5.4).

Complete surgical resection, including cytoreduction and hyperthermic intraperitoneal chemotherapy (HIPEC) for carcinomatosis, is standard therapy for appendical carcinoma and pseudomyxoma peritonei, among others [9–16]. Complete cytoreduction and HIPEC have been found to improve survival in many studies of carcinomatosis [14, 18–20]. Intraperitoneal therapy is currently the recommended approach in carcinomatosis of ovarian and mesothelioma origin [2, 17–23]. In the context of a prospective randomized trial, gastric cancer patients with

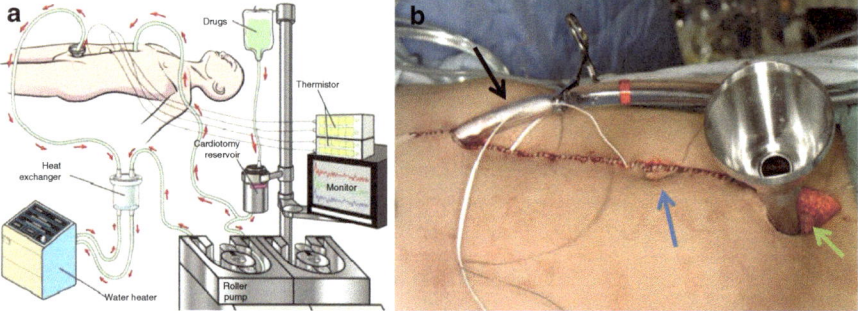

Fig. 5.4 (**a**) A representation of the HIPEC technique with a simple pump that pumps the heated chemotherapy into the abdominal cavity and recirculates, in a closed technique, over 90 min in the operating room, using cisplatin for chemotherapy in the case of DSRCT. (**b**) The closed abdomen of a patient after cytoreduction, ready to begin HIPEC. Temperature probes can be seen exiting from the midline skin closure that will be attached to a computer to provide a constant monitoring of the intra-abdominal temperature. *Black arrow* denotes inflow catheter, *green arrow* is outflow port, and *blue arrow* is the umbilicus of a supine patient

carcinomatosis underwent cytoreduction accompanied by normothermic or hyperthermic mitomycin C. The overall 5-year survival of surgery alone, normothermic, or hyperthermic perfusion was 42%, 43%, and 61%, respectively [2]. In ovarian carcinoma, significantly superior survival has been found in the intraperitoneal chemotherapy group compared to intravenous cisplatin and paclitaxel in a national prospective randomized trial [23].

This same principle was applied in the initial study of HIPEC in DSRCT. In the past, when evaluating a patient with DSRCT, surgeons were reluctant to offer surgical resection in the "face" of enormous disease burden in the abdomen and no known hope for disease control or cure. As in carcinomatosis, for sarcomatosis, HIPEC can provide control of microscopic disease in DSRCT after resection of 100% of gross disease. A phase 1 clinical trial of HIPEC in pediatric patients was completed. This trial demonstrated safety of HIPEC in children using cisplatin. The maximum tolerated dose (MTD) was 100 mg/m^2 with the dose-limiting toxicity (DLT) being grade 3 renal failure [24]. The addition of HIPEC has been used in DSRCT for effective local control. In a cohort of 26 DSRCT patients, who underwent surgical resection and HIPEC after neoadjuvant chemotherapy, the completeness of cytoreduction determined outcome. Median survival of only 26 months was reached when incomplete resection was accompanied by HIPEC compared to 63 months, with complete resection [25].

Recently, results from a phase 2 study of HIPEC in 20 pediatric sarcoma patients, including DSRCT, revealed superior survival results for patients with DSRCT compared to other sarcoma histologies. One-year survival for DSRCT patients was 93%, compared to 67% for other histologies ($p = 0.0073$). DSRCT patients had an 80% 30-month overall survival compared to children with other sarcoma histologies whom all succumbed by 15 months post-HIPEC [26]. There were no perioperative mortalities and no reoperations ("take backs"). Transient leukopenia or thrombocytopenia was seen in 15% of patients. Thirty-five percent of patients experienced serious complications including wound infections requiring drainage, urinary tract infections, and enterocutaneous fistula (in patients treated with abdominal radiation prior to HIPEC). (Operating time averages about 12 h.)

The technique of cytoreduction, decision for cytoreduction and HIPEC in DSRCT, is different from that done for adults with carcinomatosis. DSRCT is much more nodular and much less infiltrative than carcinoma, particularly in the area of the small bowel mesentery and pelvis. Dissection of tumors from the jejunal and ileal mesentery peritoneum is most often possible and can be complete without small bowel resection. Also, what can appear to be pelvic tumor-encasing ureters can be dissected free of the ureter, bladder, and rectum in most circumstances (Fig. 5.5). This is usually not the case in carcinomas [27].

In summary, DSRCT is a unique type of sarcoma for which improvements in treatment strategies are being made that have resulted in longer survival. Chemotherapy treatment should be offered despite what may be extensive disease on imaging, since aggressive surgery to completely extirpate the disease is possible, if there is a response to chemotherapy.

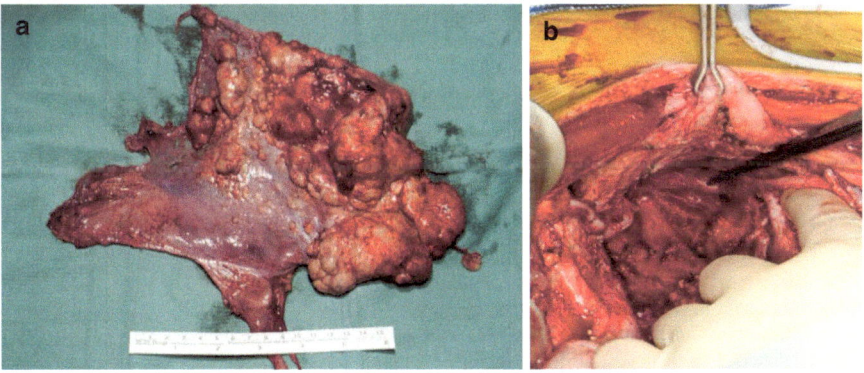

Fig. 5.5 (**a**) Pelvic peritonectomy in an 11-year-old male. (**b**) Appearance of pelvis after peritonectomy, demonstrating bladder, ureters, and vas deferens spared down to the seminal vesicles

References

1. Gerald WL, Ladanyi M, de Alava E, Cuatrecasas M, Kushner BH, LaQuaglia MP, et al. Clinical, pathologic, and molecular spectrum of tumors associated with t(11;22)(p13;q12): desmoplastic small round-cell tumor and its variants. J Clin Oncol. 1998;16(9):3028–36.
2. Park BJ, Alexander HR, Libutti SK, Wu P, Royalty D, Kranda KC, et al. Treatment of primary peritoneal mesothelioma by continuous hyperthermic peritoneal perfusion (CHPP). Ann Surg Oncol. 1999;6(6):582–90.
3. Ladanyi M, Gerald W. Fusion of the EWS and WT1 genes in the desmoplastic small round cell tumor. Cancer Res. 1994;54(11):2837–40.
4. Arnold MA, Schoenfield L, Limketkai BN, Arnold CA. Diagnostic pitfalls of differentiating desmoplastic small round cell tumor (DSRCT) from Wilms tumor (WT): overlapping morphologic and immunohistochemical features. Am J Surg Pathol. 2014;38(9):1220–6.
5. Lal DR, Su WT, Wolden SL, Loh KC, Modak S, La Quaglia MP. Results of multimodal treatment for desmoplastic small round cell tumors. J Pediatr Surg. 2005;40(1):251–5.
6. Zhang WD, Li CX, Liu QY, Hu YY, Cao Y, Huang JH. CT, MRI, and FDG-PET/CT imaging findings of abdominopelvic desmoplastic small round cell tumors: correlation with histopathologic findings. Eur J Radiol. 2010;80:269–73.
7. Kushner BH, LaQuaglia MP, Wollner N, Meyers PA, Lindsley KL, Ghavimi F, et al. Desmoplastic small round-cell tumor: prolonged progression-free survival with aggressive multimodality therapy. J Clin Oncol. 1996;14(5):1526–31.
8. Aguilera D, Hayes-Jordan A, Anderson P, Woo S, Pearson M, Green H. Outpatient and home chemotherapy with novel local control strategies in desmoplastic small round cell tumor. Sarcoma. 2008;2008:261589.
9. Glehen O, Kwiatkowski F, Sugarbaker PH, Elias D, Levine EA, De Simone M, et al. Cytoreductive surgery combined with perioperative intraperitoneal chemotherapy for the management of peritoneal carcinomatosis from colorectal cancer: a multi-institutional study. J Clin Oncol. 2004;22(16):3284–92.
10. Sugarbaker PH. A curative approach to peritoneal carcinomatosis from colorectal cancer. Semin Oncol. 2005;32(6 Suppl 9):S68–73.
11. Sugarbaker PH, Stuart OA, Yoo D. Strategies for management of the peritoneal surface component of cancer: cytoreductive surgery plus perioperative intraperitoneal chemotherapy. J Oncol Pharm Pract. 2005;11(3):111–9.
12. Sugarbaker PH, Jablonski KA. Prognostic features of 51 colorectal and 130 appendiceal cancer patients with peritoneal carcinomatosis treated by cytoreductive surgery and intraperitoneal chemotherapy. Ann Surg. 1995;221(2):124–32.
13. Glehen O, Gilly FN, Sugarbaker PH. New perspectives in the management of colorectal cancer: what about peritoneal carcinomatosis? Scand J Surg. 2003;92(2):178–9.
14. Gough DB, Donohue JH, Schutt AJ, Gonchoroff N, Goellner JR, Wilson TO, et al. Pseudomyxoma peritonei. Long-term patient survival with an aggressive regional approach. Ann Surg. 1994;219(2):112–9.
15. Sugarbaker PH, Welch LS, Mohamed F, Glehen O. A review of peritoneal mesothelioma at the Washington Cancer Institute. Surg Oncol Clin N Am. 2003;12(3):605–21. xi
16. Glehen O, Mithieux F, Osinsky D, Beaujard AC, Freyer G, Guertsch P, et al. Surgery combined with peritonectomy procedures and intraperitoneal chemohyperthermia in abdominal cancers with peritoneal carcinomatosis: a phase II study. J Clin Oncol. 2003;21(5):799–806.
17. Yan TD, Edwards G, Alderman R, Marquardt CE, Sugarbaker PH. Morbidity and mortality assessment of cytoreductive surgery and perioperative intraperitoneal chemotherapy for diffuse malignant peritoneal mesothelioma – a prospective study of 70 consecutive cases. Ann Surg Oncol. 2007;14(2):515–25.

18. Yan TD, Welch L, Black D, Sugarbaker PH. A systematic review on the efficacy of cytoreductive surgery combined with perioperative intraperitoneal chemotherapy for diffuse malignancy peritoneal mesothelioma. Ann Oncol. 2007;18(5):827–34.
19. de Bree E, Romanos J, Michalakis J, Relakis K, Georgoulias V, Melissas J, et al. Intraoperative hyperthermic intraperitoneal chemotherapy with docetaxel as second-line treatment for peritoneal carcinomatosis of gynaecological origin. Anticancer Res. 2003;23(3C):3019–27.
20. Sugarbaker PH, Alderman R, Edwards G, Marquardt CE, Gushchin V, Esquivel J, et al. Prospective morbidity and mortality assessment of cytoreductive surgery plus perioperative intraperitoneal chemotherapy to treat peritoneal dissemination of appendiceal mucinous malignancy. Ann Surg Oncol. 2006;13(5):635–44.
21. Farma JM, Pingpank JF, Libutti SK, Bartlett DL, Ohl S, Beresneva T, et al. Limited survival in patients with carcinomatosis from foregut malignancies after cytoreduction and continuous hyperthermic peritoneal perfusion. J Gastrointest Surg. 2005;9(9):1346–53.
22. Kunisaki C, Shimada H, Akiyama H, Nomura M, Matsuda G, Otsuka Y, et al. Therapeutic outcomes of continuous hyperthermic peritoneal perfusion against advanced gastric cancer with peritoneal carcinomatosis. Hepatogastroenterology. 2006;53(69):473–8.
23. Feldman AL, Libutti SK, Pingpank JF, Bartlett DL, Beresnev TH, Mavroukakis SM, et al. Analysis of factors associated with outcome in patients with malignant peritoneal mesothelioma undergoing surgical debulking and intraperitoneal chemotherapy. J Clin Oncol. 2003;21(24):4560–7.
24. Hayes-Jordan A, Green H, Ludwig J, Anderson P. Toxicity of hyperthermic intraperitoneal chemotherapy (HIPEC) in pediatric patients with sarcomatosis/carcinomatosis: early experience and phase 1 results. Pediatr Blood Cancer. 2012;59(2):395–7.
25. Hayes-Jordan A, Green HL, Lin H, Owusu-Agyemang P, Fitzgerald N, Arunkumar R, et al. Complete cytoreduction and HIPEC improves survival in desmoplastic small round cell tumor. Ann Surg Oncol. 2014;21(1):220–4.
26. Hayes-Jordan A, Green H, Xiao LC, Fournier K, Huh W, Herzog C, Ludwig J, McAleer M, Anderson P, editors. Desmoplastic small round cell tumor treated with cytoreductive surgery and hyperthermic intraperitoneal chemotherapy: results of a phase 2 trial [abstract]. American Pediatric Surgical Association Annual Meeting; 2015 April 30-May 3; Fort Lauderdale, FL.
27. Hayes-Jordan A, Green H, Lin H, Owusu-Agyemang P, Mejia R, Okhuysen-Cawley R, et al. Cytoreductive surgery and Hyperthermic Intraperitoneal Chemotherapy (HIPEC) for children, adolescents, and young adults: the first 50 cases. Ann Surg Oncol. 2015;22(5):1726–32.

Chapter 6
Peritoneal Metastasis of Retroperitoneal Tumors

Andreas Brandl, Christina Barbara Schäfer, and Beate Rau

6.1 Introduction

Peritoneal metastases of retroperitoneal tumors are in general rare. Peritoneal metastases can arise as synchronous peritoneal seeding of the primary tumor, e.g., colorectal carcinoma or pancreas carcinoma or as a tumor recurrence after surgery affecting the peritoneum, e.g., liposarcoma or leiomyosarcoma. The mechanisms for the development of peritoneal metastases are not completely understood. Cell shedding from the primary tumor is thought to be responsible for these peritoneal deposits, which may occur spontaneously or as a result of spillage during surgical procedures.

Retroperitoneal tumors can be divided in primary retroperitoneal neoplasms and primary tumors of retroperitoneal organs.

6.2 Primary Retroperitoneal Neoplasms

Primary retroperitoneal neoplasms are an extremely rare group of tumors. Due to their location and relatively unhindered growth where symptoms develop late, the size at presentation tends to be extremely large (average size 11–20 cm).

The retroperitoneum in the abdomen is the space between the posterior parietal peritoneum anteriorly and the transversalis fascia posteriorly. It extends from the diaphragm superiorly to continue into the extraperitoneal space in the pelvis inferiorly. The retroperitoneum is loosely divided into the anterior and posterior pararenal, perirenal, and great vessel spaces. The anterior pararenal space is bordered between

A. Brandl • C.B. Schäfer • B. Rau, MD, PhD (✉)
Department of General, Visceral and Transplantation Surgery and Department of General, Visceral, Vascular and Thoracic Surgery, Campus Virchow and Mitte, Charité, Universitätsmedizin Berlin, Charitéplatz 1, 10117, Berlin, Germany
e-mail: Beate.Rau@charite.de

© Springer International Publishing AG 2017
E. Canbay (ed.), *Unusual Cases in Peritoneal Surface Malignancies*,
DOI 10.1007/978-3-319-51523-6_6

the posterior parietal peritoneum anteriorly, the anterior renal or Gerota fascia posteriorly, and laterally by the lateroconal fascia. This space includes the pancreaticoduodenal space and the pericolonic space. The posterior pararenal space lies between the posterior renal fascia and the transversalis fascia, whereas the perirenal space is located between the anterior and the posterior renal fascia. The great vessel space surrounds the aorta and the inferior vena cava and is anterior to the vertebral bodies and psoas muscles. The anterior and posterior pararenal spaces merge inferior to the level of the kidneys, which communicates inferiorly with the prevesical space and extraperitoneal compartments of the pelvis [1].

Primary retroperitoneal neoplasms are a rare but an important group of neoplasms. They account for only 0.1–0.2% of all malignancies and arise outside the retroperitoneal organs [2]. Most primary retroperitoneal neoplasms develop from the mesodermal system. Liposarcoma, leiomyosarcoma, and malignant fibrous histiocytoma are responsible for more than 80% of primary retroperitoneal sarcomas. The remaining primary retroperitoneal masses arise predominantly from the nervous system [1].

Owing to the loose connective tissue of the retroperitoneum, these masses tend to be large (11–20 cm) at the time of presentation [1]. They can be identified incidentally or may present clinically with a palpable abdominal or pelvic mass. Cross-sectional imaging has revolutionized the investigation of patients with retroperitoneal neoplasms. Both CT and MRI scan play an integral role in the characterization of these masses and in evaluation of their extent and involvement of adjacent structures and therefore in treatment planning.

6.3 Primary Tumors of Retroperitoneal Organs

The classification of retroperitoneal organs divides primary and secondary retroperitoneal organs due to the embryonic development. The characteristic between them is that secondary retroperitoneal organs lost their mesentery during development, while the primary retroperitoneal organs never had a mesentery.

Major primary retroperitoneal organs are:

• Kidneys
• Adrenal glands
• Ureters
• Aorta
• Inferior vena cava
• Lower rectum

Major secondary retroperitoneal organs are:

• Duodenum (descending and horizontal part)
• Pancreas (head, neck, and body)

- Ascending colon
- Descending colon
- Upper rectum

Most of the tumors of retroperitoneal organs are diagnosed by CT or MRI scan or by endoscopy.

6.4   Peritoneal Metastases and Treatment

6.4.1   Primary Retroperitoneal Tumors

Peritoneal metastases of primary retroperitoneal tumors are rare, and most of them occur as implant metastases described as local recurrence after surgical procedures.

6.4.1.1   Liposarcoma

Soft tissue sarcomas are rare mesenchymal tumors, accounting for 1% of all adult solid malignancies. Up to 30% of soft tissue sarcomas arise in the abdominopelvic cavity or the retroperitoneum. Retroperitoneal and both gastrointestinal and gynecological visceral sarcoma are associated with high rates of local–regional relapse after surgical resection, due to anatomical and biological features. Peritoneal sarcomatosis refers to a condition in which the intraabdominal soft tissue sarcoma spread is the dominant clinical picture. It may occur at first presentation or more often at the final stage of disease progression, especially when the primary tumor has been ruptured spontaneously or surgically [3, 4].

Peritoneal sarcomatosis has traditionally been viewed as a terminal disease with a median survival of less than 1 year, with surgery only reserved for associated complications such as intestinal obstruction and ureteral obstruction [4–6]. Bilimoria et al. found the median survival of patients with sarcomatosis treated with palliative surgery and/or chemotherapy to be 13 months with the only negative prognostic factor being tumor volume [4]. This result is in line with other published reports describing the experience with palliation that have found the median survival to range from 7 to 15 months [5, 6].

The addition of intraperitoneal chemotherapy to cytoreductive surgery (CRS) has not been shown to improve on the results achieved with CRS alone and is therefore currently not recommended in the treatment of sarcomatosis except in well-selected patients with low tumor burden after complete cytoreduction and as part of an experimental protocol preferably in centers with expertise in peritonectomy procedures using hyperthermic intraperitoneal chemotherapy (HIPEC) as the intraperitoneal chemotherapy modality [7].

6.4.1.2   Leiomyosarcoma

It is an uncommon malignant neoplasm of smooth muscle origin that tends to arise in the retroperitoneum, peripheral soft tissues, genitourinary tract, gastrointestinal tract, and large vessels and rarely in bones [8]. About 20–67% of cases of leiomyosarcoma develop in the retroperitoneum. Complete surgical resection with wide margins reduces the rate of local recurrence; however, in retroperitoneum, it is difficult to procure wide margins all the way around the tumor due to the major vessels and other important structures [8]. Even when complete excision is believed to have been accomplished, local recurrence rates are as high as 40–77% [9]. Leiomyosarcomas have propensity for hematogenous spread and infrequently metastasize to lymph nodes. Distant metastases are present at the time of diagnosis in approximately 40% of cases, and most patients who survive the primary tumor will eventually develop metastases [9]. The liver and lungs are the most common sites of metastasis in patients with leiomyosarcoma [8, 10]. Other manifestations of tumor spread include mesenteric or omental metastases, retroperitoneal lymphadenopathy, soft tissue metastases, bone metastases, splenic metastases, and ascites.

Among leiomyosarcomas of all sites, the retroperitoneal leiomyosarcomas have the worst prognosis, and about 80–87% of these patients die within 5 years [9]. Cure of the primary tumor is difficult because of late presentation, origin within deep tissue, inability to achieve wide surgical margins, and relative insensitivity to chemotherapy and radiotherapy [8, 9]. Single or few metastatic lesions have been surgically treated in various reports [11, 12].

There is no data about the effect of CRS and HIPEC in patients suffering from leiomyosarcoma.

6.4.1.3   Malignant Fibrous Histiocytoma

Malignant fibrous histiocytoma is a typically large deep-seated tumor showing progressive, often rapid enlargement. In addition, this tumor has high propensity for metastasis to other organs, such as the lung, bone, and liver.

The treatment of malignant fibrous histiocytoma remains uncertain. Radical excision and postoperative radiotherapy are thought to control local recurrence but are limited to localized tumor [13]. When distant metastasis is seen, surgical resection with curative intention is only possible for patients with limited pulmonary metastases who are also undergoing or have undergone complete resection of the primary tumor [14]. Actually, however, surgical resections of metastatic tumors may improve quality of life and manage complications related to metastasis although they did not prove the survival benefit.

Peritoneal metastases from malignant fibrous histiocytoma are described in a case report, which reflects that this is an extremely rare metastatic site from a rare tumor [15]. Treatment options in these patients have to be assessed on an individual base. Due to the fact of only one published case, CRS and HIPEC have not been described as therapeutic options for this indication.

6.4.2   Primary Tumors of Retroperitoneal Organs

6.4.2.1   Kidney

Renal cell carcinoma spreads predominantly by direct extension, lymphatic dissemination, or venous invasion. Intraperitoneal metastatic spread of RCC involving mesentery and omentum is very uncommon.

To our knowledge, there are four case reports compiling six cases of peritoneal metastases of renal cell cancer [16–19].

The CT findings in three cases included extensive ascites, widespread omental infiltration, and peritoneal implants, as well as retroperitoneal metastases [17].

Besides the aggressive RCC subtypes with adverse histopathological features (sarcomatoid differentiation, presence of tumor necrosis, microvascular invasion and high grade), which can present with diffuse peritoneal metastases involving the omentum, also early stages of renal cell carcinoma are able to develop omental metastases after surgery [19].

The treatment of metastatic renal cancer is still controversial since large series of metastasectomies are reported in the literature, but little is known about the management of metastasis in atypical sites, like the peritoneum.

Surgical resection remains a critical mode of achieving control of long-term disease in metastatic RCC patients.

6.4.2.2   Adrenal Glands

Adrenocortical carcinoma is an aggressive but rare malignancy with an incidence of 0.5–2 cases per million per year [20–23]. Five-year survival rates vary from 16 to 40% and are largely dependent on the adrenocortical carcinoma stage at diagnosis [24].

Complete R0 resection of adrenocortical carcinoma is currently the keystone and only curative treatment modality for patients with this type of tumor. Unfortunately, ACC is a highly malignant tumor, with up to 70–85% of patients experiencing recurrence after surgical resection [25–28].

In a large national retrospective study, the best predictors of prolonged survival after first recurrence were time to first recurrence over 12 months and R0 resection. These data suggest that radical reoperation should be offered to patients with delayed recurrence [29]. In recurrent cases, a median survival of 179 days for patients who had no therapy, 226 days for patients managed without surgery, and 1,272 days for those who had debulking surgery were demonstrated [30]. Based on these data, patients with recurrent ACC may benefit from operative intervention, with improvement in survival and symptoms.

Mitotane monotherapy is indicated in the management of patients with metastatic disease with a low tumor burden or more indolent disease, whereas patients with aggressive disease need cytotoxic chemotherapy like mitotane plus either a combination of etoposide, doxorubicin, and cisplatin (EDP) every 4 weeks or streptozocin every 3 weeks [31]. This therapy is now the established first-line cytotoxic therapy.

6.4.2.3 Ureter

Peritoneal metastases from urothelial carcinoma of the ureter are rarely described. A recent study reported in 5 of 117 patients with upper urinary tract urothelial carcinoma initially treated with laparoscopic radical nephroureterectomy of peritoneal implants as atypic distant metastases [32].

Nevertheless, there is no data or recommendations about evidence-based, standardized treatment for these patients.

6.4.2.4 Aorta

Rhabdomyosarcomas of the large arteries are more common in the heart and aortic arch compared to the abdominal aorta.

To our knowledge, there is only one published case report about a rhabdomyosarcoma of the abdominal aorta. The authors report an 11-year-old boy with retroperitoneal alveolar rhabdomyosarcoma at the aortoiliac bifurcation. There is no data about peritoneal metastases of this disease so far.

6.4.2.5 Inferior Vena Cava

Primary leiomyosarcoma of the inferior vena cava is a rare neoplasia of the smooth muscle of the vein wall that accounts for approximately 0.5% of soft tissue sarcomas, with fewer than 390 cases reported in the literature [33, 34]. Surgery is the cornerstone of treatment for these tumors, but most inferior vena cava sarcomas recur even after complete resection and are associated with low disease-free survival rates [33, 35–37]. Nevertheless, good overall survival rates have previously been reported in patients treated in tertiary referral centers [33, 38].

Few publications discuss the management of recurrent inferior vena cava leiomyosarcoma. As a result, a standardized approach has not been established. Currently, surgery is the only option offered for recurrent disease if associated with minimal morbidity, even for isolated metastatic disease. The most commonly performed procedure is local excision for retroperitoneal recurrence and metastasectomy in case of lung recurrence [37, 39–44]. Adjuvant chemotherapy based on doxorubicin or a combination of doxorubicin and ifosfamide may extend the time to recurrence and increase overall survival in sarcoma patients [45, 46].

6.4.2.6 Rectum: Ascending Colon, Descending Colon

It is estimated that up to 10% of patients with colon cancer and up to 5% of patients with rectal cancer eventually develop peritoneal metastases [47, 48]. Cytoreductive surgery (CRS) followed by hyperthermic intraperitoneal chemotherapy (HIPEC) has resulted in promising survival rates with acceptable treatment-related morbidity and mortality [49, 50]. Many retrospective studies showed median overall survival rates >36 months and 5-year survival rates between 30 and 40%. Therefore, CRS and HIPEC are currently considered to be the standard of care in selected patients with colorectal peritoneal metastases in several countries [51]. The surgical treatment goal is complete cytoreduction in these patients. To achieve this goal, common selection criteria in many centers are the extent of peritoneal metastases which is evaluated with the peritoneal cancer index (PCI). This index was first introduced by Paul Sugarbaker in 1996 and ranges from 0 to 39. The score assesses the extent of disease by classifying the tumor size and the involvement of the parietal peritoneum and the small bowel.

6.4.2.7 Duodenum (Descending and Horizontal Part)

Primary duodenal tumors are generally rare diseases. The most common are the adenocarcinoma and the gastrointestinal stromal tumor (GIST) of the duodenum. GIST are mesenchymal tumors of the gastrointestinal tract. Duodenal GIST are 1–4% of all gastrointestinal stromal tumors [52]. Complete surgical resection remains the best option in the treatment of GISTs, although imatinib mesylate, a tyrosine kinase inhibitor, may be effective in c-kit-positive tumors [53, 54]. About 40% of patients with primary GISTs who undergo complete resection are reported to have recurrent disease, most recurrences being local or liver metastases with a median follow-up of 24 months [55, 56]. For duodenal GISTs, the recurrence-free survival rate at 1–3 years of follow-up following resection has been reported to be 100%, 86.7%, and 95.2%, respectively [53, 56, 57]. A good prognosis is particularly seen in those who have undergone complete resection of the tumor. However, in a series from the pre-imatinib era, Miettenen et al., while reporting on the outcome in 156 patients who had surgery for duodenal GISTs, noted local recurrence, metastasis, or both in 35% of their patients [55].

Data about peritoneal metastases or peritoneal implants are missing. Farma et al. (2005) reported in a single center study that two patients with adenocarcinoma of the duodenum in a series of foregut malignancies with peritoneal metastases were treated with optimal cytoreduction and HIPEC with cisplatin for 90 min. The median progression-free survival of the study group was 8 months (mean, 10 months; range, 1–47 months) with a median overall survival of 8 months (mean, 18 months; range, 1–74 months). They concluded that peritoneal perfusion with cisplatin used to treat foregut malignancies has a high incidence of complications and does not significantly alter the natural history of the disease [58].

6.4.2.8 Pancreas (Head, Neck, and Body)

Most patients with pancreatic cancer present with distant metastasis at diagnosis. Peritoneal carcinomatosis, which is one of the most frequently encountered modes of metastasis, can cause several burdensome manifestations such as massive ascites, intestinal obstruction, and hydronephrosis [59]. Therefore, peritoneal carcinomatosis has been regarded as a far advanced disease amenable only to palliation of symptoms because it severely impairs the quality of life of patients.

Recently, several studies reported the advancement in intervention for gastrointestinal obstruction caused by peritoneal carcinomatosis [60–62]. These palliative procedures enable to maintain performance status well and therefore promote the use of aggressive therapy even in patients with peritoneal carcinomatous [63]. As a result, multidisciplinary treatment can be a choice of treatment in patients with several types of cancer with peritoneal carcinomatosis.

A population-based study of 2,924 pancreatic cancer patients showed that synchronous peritoneal carcinomatosis was observed in 9% of all patients, and an autopsy study reported that 22% of patients who died from pancreatic cancer had developed peritoneal carcinomatosis [64, 65].

One possible option for improving the management of peritoneal carcinomatosis might be intraperitoneal chemotherapy. It has been developed to enhance antitumor activity against peritoneal metastasis by maintaining a high concentration of the administered drug in the peritoneal cavity over a long period while sparing systemic host tissues from drug toxicity. Currently, a Japanese clinical trial comparing systemic with intraperitoneal chemotherapy is ongoing for refractory pancreatic cancer with malignant ascites [66].

Schneitler et al. published a case report of one patient with peritoneal carcinomatosis and liver metastases of the pancreas cancer treated with FOLFIRINOX (consisting of 5-FU/folinic acid, irinotecan, and oxaliplatin) followed by CRS and HIPEC [67]. The follow-up of 11 months after operation proved complete oncologic remission. This therapeutic regimen might only be chosen in selected patients, while the majority of patients with peritoneal metastases of pancreatic cancer are treated with palliative chemotherapy either with FOLFIRINOX or gemcitabine monotherapy. FOLFIRONOX was reported to achieve an average life extension of 11.1 months compared to the extension of 6.8 months that was achieved using gemcitabine monotherapy [68].

6.5   Conclusion

Peritoneal metastases of retroperitoneal tumors are in general rare. Cytoreductive surgery (CRS) and hyperthermic intraperitoneal chemotherapy (HIPEC) can be an option for selected patients with colorectal cancer. The therapeutic regimen of all other tumor origins has to be individually discussed while palliative therapy is most common.

Large international databases may help to deliver more evidence for prognosis and treatment options in these rare diseases.

Funding/Support The authors have no financial relationships to disclose, neither grants, equipment, nor drugs.

Conflicts The authors have no conflict of interest to disclose.

References

1. Rajiah P, Sinha R, Cuevas C, Dubinsky TJ, Bush Jr WII, Kolokythas O. Imaging of uncommon retroperitoneal masses. Radiographics. 2011;31(4):949–76. doi:10.1148/rg.314095132.
2. Neville A, Herts BR. CT characteristics of primary retroperitoneal neoplasms. Crit Rev Comput Tomogr. 2004;45(4):247–70.
3. Karakousis CP, Blumenson LE, Canavese G, Rao U. Surgery for disseminated abdominal sarcoma. Am J Surg. 1992;163(6):560–4.
4. Bilimoria MM, Holtz DJ, Mirza NQ, Feig BW, Pisters PW, Patel S, et al. Tumor volume as a prognostic factor for sarcomatosis. Cancer. 2002;94(9):2441–6. doi:10.1002/cncr.10504.
5. Chu DZ, Lang NP, Thompson C, Osteen PK, Westbrook KC. Peritoneal carcinomatosis in nongynecologic malignancy. A prospective study of prognostic factors. Cancer. 1989;63(2):364–7.
6. Mudan SS, Conlon KC, Woodruff JM, Lewis JJ, Brennan MF. Salvage surgery for patients with recurrent gastrointestinal sarcoma: prognostic factors to guide patient selection. Cancer. 2000;88(1):66–74.
7. Munene G, Mack LA, Temple WJ. Systematic review on the efficacy of multimodal treatment of sarcomatosis with cytoreduction and intraperitoneal chemotherapy. Ann Surg Oncol. 2011;18(1):207–13. doi:10.1245/s10434-010-1229-3.
8. O'Sullivan PJ, Harris AC, Munk PL. Radiological imaging features of non-uterine leiomyosarcoma. Br J Radiol. 2008;81(961):73–81. doi:10.1259/bjr/18595145.
9. Hartman DS, Hayes WS, Choyke PL, Tibbetts GP. From the archives of the AFIP. Leiomyosarcoma of the retroperitoneum and inferior vena cava: radiologic-pathologic correlation. Radiographics. 1992;12(6):1203–20. doi:10.1148/radiographics.12.6.1439022.
10. McLeod AJ, Zornoza J, Shirkhoda A. Leiomyosarcoma: computed tomographic findings. Radiology. 1984;152(1):133–6. doi:10.1148/radiology.152.1.6729102.
11. Courtney MW, Levine EA. Uterine leiomyosarcoma metastatic to soft tissue of the flank following a ten-year disease-free interval. South Med J. 2009;102(3):325–6. doi:10.1097/SMJ.0b013e318195132a.
12. Burke JP, Maguire D, Dillon J, Moriarty M, O'Toole GC. Whipple's procedure for an oligometastasis to the pancreas from a leiomyosarcoma of the thigh. Ir J Med Sci. 2012;181(3):361–3. doi:10.1007/s11845-009-0447-9.
13. Gibbs JF, Huang PP, Lee RJ, McGrath B, Brooks J, McKinley B, et al. Malignant fibrous histiocytoma: an institutional review. Cancer Investig. 2001;19(1):23–7.
14. Putnam Jr JB, Roth JA. Surgical treatment for pulmonary metastases from sarcoma. Hematol Oncol Clin North Am. 1995;9(4):869–87.
15. Yoo JW, Lee DH, Song HJ, Ahn JH, Kim SW, Suh C, et al. Peritoneal dissemination from malignant fibrous histiocytoma of the buttock: unusual metastases from a rare tumor. Gut Liver. 2008;2(3):213–5. doi:10.5009/gnl.2008.2.3.213.
16. Stavropoulos NJ, Deliveliotis C, Kouroupakis D, Demonakou M, Kastriotis J, Dimopoulos C. Renal cell carcinoma presenting as a large abdominal mass with an extensive peritoneal metastasis. Urol Int. 1995;54(3):169–70.

17. Tartar VM, Heiken JP, McClennan BL. Renal cell carcinoma presenting with diffuse peritoneal metastases: CT findings. J Comput Assist Tomogr. 1991;15(3):450–3.
18. Staderini F, Cianchi F, Badii B, Skalamera I, Fiorenza G, Foppa C, et al. A unique presentation of a renal clear cell carcinoma with atypical metastases. Int J Surg Case Rep. 2015;11:29–32. doi:10.1016/j.ijscr.2015.03.009.
19. Acar O, Mut T, Saglican Y, Sag AA, Falay O, Selcukbiricik F, et al. Isolated omental metastasis of renal cell carcinoma after extraperitoneal open partial nephrectomy: a case report. Int J Surg Case Rep. 2016;21:6–11. doi:10.1016/j.ijscr.2016.02.008.
20. Kebebew E, Reiff E, Duh QY, Clark OH, McMillan A. Extent of disease at presentation and outcome for adrenocortical carcinoma: have we made progress? World J Surg. 2006;30(5):872–8. doi:10.1007/s00268-005-0329-x.
21. Golden SH, Robinson KA, Saldanha I, Anton B, Ladenson PW. Clinical review: prevalence and incidence of endocrine and metabolic disorders in the United States: a comprehensive review. J Clin Endocrinol Metab. 2009;94(6):1853–78. doi:10.1210/jc.2008-2291.
22. Fassnacht M, Kroiss M, Allolio B. Update in adrenocortical carcinoma. J Clin Endocrinol Metab. 2013;98(12):4551–64. doi:10.1210/jc.2013-3020.
23. Kerkhofs TM, Verhoeven RH, Van der Zwan JM, Dieleman J, Kerstens MN, Links TP, et al. Adrenocortical carcinoma: a population-based study on incidence and survival in the Netherlands since 1993. Eur J Cancer. 2013;49(11):2579–86. doi:10.1016/j.ejca.2013.02.034.
24. Fassnacht M, Johanssen S, Quinkler M, Bucsky P, Willenberg HS, Beuschlein F, et al. Limited prognostic value of the 2004 international union against cancer staging classification for adrenocortical carcinoma: proposal for a revised TNM classification. Cancer. 2009;115(2):243–50. doi:10.1002/cncr.24030.
25. Terzolo M, Baudin AE, Ardito A, Kroiss M, Leboulleux S, Daffara F, et al. Mitotane levels predict the outcome of patients with adrenocortical carcinoma treated adjuvantly following radical resection. Eur J Endocrinol. 2013;169(3):263–70. doi:10.1530/EJE-13-0242.
26. Gratian L, Pura J, Dinan M, Reed S, Scheri R, Roman S, et al. Treatment patterns and outcomes for patients with adrenocortical carcinoma associated with hospital case volume in the United States. Ann Surg Oncol. 2014;21(11):3509–14. doi:10.1245/s10434-014-3931-z.
27. Stojadinovic A, Brennan MF, Hoos A, Omeroglu A, Leung DH, Dudas ME, et al. Adrenocortical adenoma and carcinoma: histopathological and molecular comparative analysis. Mod Pathol. 2003;16(8):742–51. doi:10.1097/01.MP.0000081730.72305.81.
28. Kerkhofs TM, Verhoeven RH, Bonjer HJ, van Dijkum EJ, Vriens MR, De Vries J, et al. Surgery for adrenocortical carcinoma in The Netherlands: analysis of the national cancer registry data. Eur J Endocrinol. 2013;169(1):83–9. doi:10.1530/EJE-13-0142.
29. Erdogan I, Deutschbein T, Jurowich C, Kroiss M, Ronchi C, Quinkler M, et al. The role of surgery in the management of recurrent adrenocortical carcinoma. J Clin Endocrinol Metab. 2013;98(1):181–91. doi:10.1210/jc.2012-2559.
30. Dy BM, Wise KB, Richards ML, Young Jr WF, Grant CS, Bible KC, et al. Operative intervention for recurrent adrenocortical cancer. Surgery. 2013;154(6):1292–9. discussion 9 doi:10.1016/j.surg.2013.06.033.
31. Fassnacht M, Terzolo M, Allolio B, Baudin E, Haak H, Berruti A, et al. Combination chemotherapy in advanced adrenocortical carcinoma. N Engl J Med. 2012;366(23):2189–97. doi:10.1056/NEJMoa1200966.
32. Carrion A, Huguet J, Garcia-Cruz E, Izquierdo L, Mateu L, Musquera M, et al. Intraoperative prognostic factors and atypical patterns of recurrence in patients with upper urinary tract urothelial carcinoma treated with laparoscopic radical nephroureterectomy. Scand J Urol. 2016:1–8. doi:10.3109/21681805.2016.1144219.
33. Hollenbeck ST, Grobmyer SR, Kent KC, Brennan MF. Surgical treatment and outcomes of patients with primary inferior vena cava leiomyosarcoma. J Am Coll Surg. 2003;197(4):575–9. doi:10.1016/S1072-7515(03)00433-2.
34. Wachtel H, Gupta M, Bartlett EK, Jackson BM, Kelz RR, Karakousis GC, et al. Outcomes after resection of leiomyosarcomas of the inferior vena cava: a pooled data analysis of 377 cases. Surg Oncol. 2015;24(1):21–7. doi:10.1016/j.suronc.2014.10.007.

35. Mingoli A, Cavallaro A, Sapienza P, Di Marzo L, Feldhaus RJ, Cavallari N. International registry of inferior vena cava leiomyosarcoma: analysis of a world series on 218 patients. Anticancer Res. 1996;16(5B):3201–5.
36. Ito H, Hornick JL, Bertagnolli MM, George S, Morgan JA, Baldini EH, et al. Leiomyosarcoma of the inferior vena cava: survival after aggressive management. Ann Surg Oncol. 2007;14(12):3534–41. doi:10.1245/s10434-007-9552-z.
37. Kieffer E, Alaoui M, Piette JC, Cacoub P, Chiche L. Leiomyosarcoma of the inferior vena cava: experience in 22 cases. Ann Surg. 2006;244(2):289–95. doi:10.1097/01. sla.0000229964.71743.db.
38. Wachtel H, Jackson BM, Bartlett EK, Karakousis GC, Roses RE, Bavaria JE, et al. Resection of primary leiomyosarcoma of the inferior vena cava (IVC) with reconstruction: a case series and review of the literature. J Surg Oncol. 2015;111(3):328–33. doi:10.1002/jso.23798.
39. Illum.....inati G, Calio FG, D'Urso A, Giacobbi D, Papaspyropoulos V, Ceccanei G. Prosthetic replacement of the infrahepatic inferior vena cava for leiomyosarcoma. Arch Surg. 2006;141(9):919–24. discussion 24 doi:10.1001/archsurg.141.9.919.
40. Daylami R, Amiri A, Goldsmith B, Troppmann C, Schneider PD, Khatri VP. Inferior vena cava leiomyosarcoma: is reconstruction necessary after resection? J Am Coll Surg. 2010;210(2):185–90. doi:10.1016/j.jamcollsurg.2009.10.010.
41. Mann GN, Mann LV, Levine EA, Shen P. Primary leiomyosarcoma of the inferior vena cava: a 2-institution analysis of outcomes. Surgery. 2012;151(2):261–7. doi:10.1016/j. surg.2010.10.011.
42. Cho SW, Marsh JW, Geller DA, Holtzman M, Zeh 3rd H, Bartlett DL, et al. Surgical management of leiomyosarcoma of the inferior vena cava. J Gastrointest Surg. 2008;12(12):2141–8. doi:10.1007/s11605-008-0700-y.
43. Benjamin RS, Legha SS, Patel SR, Nicaise C. Single-agent ifosfamide studies in sarcomas of soft tissue and bone: the M.D. Anderson experience. Cancer Chemother Pharmacol. 1993;31(Suppl 2):S174–9.
44. Le Cesne A, Antoine E, Spielmann M, Le Chevalier T, Brain E, Toussaint C, et al. High-dose ifosfamide: circumvention of resistance to standard-dose ifosfamide in advanced soft tissue sarcomas. J Clin Oncol. 1995;13(7):1600–8.
45. Kim JT, Kwon T, Cho Y, Shin S, Lee S, Moon D. Multidisciplinary treatment and long-term outcomes in six patients with leiomyosarcoma of the inferior vena cava. J Korean Surg Soc. 2012;82(2):101–9. doi:10.4174/jkss.2012.82.2.101.
46. Gronchi A, Miceli R, Allard MA, Callegaro D, Le Pechoux C, Fiore M, et al. Personalizing the approach to retroperitoneal soft tissue sarcoma: histology-specific patterns of failure and postrelapse outcome after primary extended resection. Ann Surg Oncol. 2015;22(5):1447–54. doi:10.1245/s10434-014-4130-7.
47. Lemmens VE, Klaver YL, Verwaal VJ, Rutten HJ, Coebergh JW, de Hingh IH. Predictors and survival of synchronous peritoneal carcinomatosis of colorectal origin: a population-based study. Int J Cancer. 2011;128(11):2717–25. doi:10.1002/ijc.25596.
48. Segelman J, Granath F, Holm T, Machado M, Mahteme H, Martling A. Incidence, prevalence and risk factors for peritoneal carcinomatosis from colorectal cancer. Br J Surg. 2012;99(5):699–705. doi:10.1002/bjs.8679.
49. Glehen O, Gilly FN, Boutitie F, Bereder JM, Quenet F, Sideris L, et al. Toward curative treatment of peritoneal carcinomatosis from nonovarian origin by cytoreductive surgery combined with perioperative intraperitoneal chemotherapy: a multi-institutional study of 1,290 patients. Cancer. 2010;116(24):5608–18. doi:10.1002/cncr.25356.
50. Kuijpers AM, Mirck B, Aalbers AG, Nienhuijs SW, de Hingh IH, Wiezer MJ, et al. Cytoreduction and HIPEC in the Netherlands: nationwide long-term outcome following the Dutch protocol. Ann Surg Oncol. 2013;20(13):4224–30. doi:10.1245/s10434-013-3145-9.
51. Esquivel J, Piso P, Verwaal V, Bachleitner-Hofmann T, Glehen O, Gonzalez-Moreno S, et al. American Society of Peritoneal Surface Malignancies opinion statement on defining expectations from cytoreductive surgery and hyperthermic intraperitoneal chemotherapy in patients with colorectal cancer. J Surg Oncol. 2014;110(7):777–8. doi:10.1002/jso.23722.

52. Meesters B, Pauwels PA, Pijnenburg AM, Vlasveld LT, Repelaer van Driel OJ. Metastasis in a benign duodenal stromal tumour. Eur J Surg Oncol. 1998;24(4):334–5.
53. Chung JC, Chu CW, Cho GS, Shin EJ, Lim CW, Kim HC, et al. Management and outcome of gastrointestinal stromal tumors of the duodenum. J Gastrointest Surg. 2010;14(5):880–3. doi:10.1007/s11605-010-1170-6.
54. Cohen MH, Cortazar P, Justice R, Pazdur R. Approval summary: imatinib mesylate in the adjuvant treatment of malignant gastrointestinal stromal tumors. Oncologist. 2010;15(3):300–7. doi:10.1634/theoncologist.2009-0120.
55. Miettinen M, Kopczynski J, Makhlouf HR, Sarlomo-Rikala M, Gyorffy H, Burke A, et al. Gastrointestinal stromal tumors, intramural leiomyomas, and leiomyosarcomas in the duodenum: a clinicopathologic, immunohistochemical, and molecular genetic study of 167 cases. Am J Surg Pathol. 2003;27(5):625–41.
56. Gervaz P, Huber O, Morel P. Surgical management of gastrointestinal stromal tumours. Br J Surg. 2009;96(6):567–78. doi:10.1002/bjs.6601.
57. Bucher P, Egger JF, Gervaz P, Ris F, Weintraub D, Villiger P, et al. An audit of surgical management of gastrointestinal stromal tumours (GIST). Eur J Surg Oncol. 2006;32(3):310–4. doi:10.1016/j.ejso.2005.11.021.
58. Farma JM, Pingpank JF, Libutti SK, Bartlett DL, Ohl S, Beresneva T, et al. Limited survival in patients with carcinomatosis from foregut malignancies after cytoreduction and continuous hyperthermic peritoneal perfusion. J Gastrointest Surg. 2005;9(9):1346–53. doi:10.1016/j.gassur.2005.06.016.
59. Sadeghi B, Arvieux C, Glehen O, Beaujard AC, Rivoire M, Baulieux J, et al. Peritoneal carcinomatosis from non-gynecologic malignancies: results of the EVOCAPE 1 multicentric prospective study. Cancer. 2000;88(2):358–63.
60. Isayama H, Sasaki T, Nakai Y, Togawa O, Kogure H, Sasahira N, et al. Management of malignant gastric outlet obstruction with a modified triple-layer covered metal stent. Gastrointest Endosc. 2012;75(4):757–63. doi:10.1016/j.gie.2011.11.035.
61. Sasaki T, Isayama H, Nakai Y, Togawa O, Kogure H, Kawakubo K, et al. Predictive factors of solid food intake in patients with malignant gastric outlet obstruction receiving self-expandable metallic stents for palliation. Dig Endosc. 2012;24(4):226–30. doi:10.1111/j.1443-1661.2011.01208.x.
62. Sasaki T, Isayama H, Maetani I, Nakai Y, Kogure H, Kawakubo K, et al. Japanese multicenter estimation of WallFlex duodenal stent for unresectable malignant gastric outlet obstruction. Dig Endosc. 2013;25(1):1–6. doi:10.1111/j.1443-1661.2012.01319.x.
63. Nakai Y, Ishigami H, Isayama H, Sasaki T, Kawakubo K, Kogure H, et al. Role of intervention for biliary and gastric/intestinal obstruction in gastric cancer with peritoneal metastasis. J Gastroenterol Hepatol. 2012;27(12):1796–800. doi:10.1111/j.1440-1746.2012.07241.x.
64. Thomassen I, Lemmens VE, Nienhuijs SW, Luyer MD, Klaver YL, de Hingh IH. Incidence, prognosis, and possible treatment strategies of peritoneal carcinomatosis of pancreatic origin: a population-based study. Pancreas. 2013;42(1):72–5. doi:10.1097/MPA.0b013e31825abf8c.
65. Blastik M, Plavecz E, Zalatnai A. Pancreatic carcinomas in a 60-year, institute-based autopsy material with special emphasis of metastatic pattern. Pancreas. 2011;40(3):478–80. doi:10.1097/MPA.0b013e318205e332.
66. Takahara N, Isayama H, Nakai Y, Sasaki T, Ishigami H, Yamashita H, et al. Intravenous and intraperitoneal paclitaxel with S-1 for refractory pancreatic cancer with malignant ascites: an interim analysis. J Gastrointest Cancer. 2014;45(3):307–11. doi:10.1007/s12029-014-9603-1.
67. Schneitler S, Kropil P, Riemer J, Antoch G, Knoefel WT, Haussinger D, et al. Metastasized pancreatic carcinoma with neoadjuvant FOLFIRINOX therapy and R0 resection. World J Gastroenterol. 2015;21(20):6384–90. doi:10.3748/wjg.v21.i20.6384.
68. Conroy T, Desseigne F, Ychou M, Bouche O, Guimbaud R, Becouarn Y, et al. FOLFIRINOX versus gemcitabine for metastatic pancreatic cancer. N Engl J Med. 2011;364(19):1817–25. doi:10.1056/NEJMoa1011923.

Chapter 7
Management of Peritoneal Metastasis from Uterine Sarcoma

Carlos A. Muñoz-Zuluaga, Arkadii Sipok, and Armando Sardi

7.1 Introduction

Uterine sarcomas (US) are a group of rare heterogeneous mesenchymal malignancies arising from uterine stromal musculature or connective tissue [1]. US represent only 1% of all female genital malignancies and 3–9% of uterine tumors [2]. Over the past decade, the incidence of tumors from the uterine corpus has been rising, making up 60,050 (20%) of new cases of all female genital tract tumors reported in the United States in 2016 [3]. Risk factors are difficult to estimate, due to the rarity of the disease. However, it is generally accepted that race (African descent) [4, 5], chronic tamoxifen usage (>5 years) [6, 7], and inherited syndromes and conditions (hereditary leiomyomatosis, renal cell carcinoma, and retinoblastoma) increase the risk of developing US [8, 9].

Peritoneal sarcomatosis (PS) is a rare condition that presents as an aggressive tumor involving the peritoneum. This may develop after removing the uterus laparoscopically, transabdominally, or vaginally for benign or malignant conditions and is characterized by vague, nonspecific symptoms often leading to a delay in diagnosis and, as a result, poor prognosis [10 12]. Treatment outcomes depend on tumor size, histopathological type, and stage [13]. Patients with PS from leiomyosarcoma (LMS) reportedly have an overall survival (OS) of only 27 months [14]. Survival from high-grade endometrial stromal sarcoma ranges between 17 and 53 months, while low-grade endometrial stromal sarcomas have significantly better survival at more than 80 months [14–16].

Patients with disseminated US who are treated with optimal cytoreductive surgery alone have a median OS of 23–29 months, with a 5-year survival from 4% to 37% [17, 18]. Treatment with systemic chemotherapy has a reported median overall

C.A. Muñoz-Zuluaga • A. Sipok • A. Sardi (✉)
Institute for Cancer Care, Mercy Medical Center, Baltimore, MD, USA
e-mail: asardi@mdmercy.com

© Springer International Publishing AG 2017
E. Canbay (ed.), *Unusual Cases in Peritoneal Surface Malignancies*,
DOI 10.1007/978-3-319-51523-6_7

survival of 15–18 months when using gemcitabine plus docetaxel as first-line agents, with median progression-free survival of 4–6 months [19, 20].

To date, there is no standard of care treatment for peritoneal dissemination of US. Treatment generally involves cytoreductive surgery (CRS) with systemic chemotherapy for palliation, resulting in relatively poor outcomes [21]. In an attempt to improve patient survival, while reducing intraperitoneal recurrences, CRS, combined with hyperthermic intraperitoneal chemotherapy (HIPEC), has been used as a treatment modality and has demonstrated promising results with a 5-year survival of 65% [11, 12, 22–24].

7.2 Histopathology

According to the 2014 World Health Organization (WHO) classification, uterine corpus tumors are classified into six categories: epithelial and precursors, mesenchymal, mixed epithelial and mesenchymal, miscellaneous, lymphoid, and secondary tumors [25]. US appear in the mesenchymal and mixed epithelial and mesenchymal groups since they arise from uterine musculature or connective tissue and are characterized by malignant behavior [1]. The main histopathological subtypes are depicted in Fig. 7.1.

Carcinosarcoma (CS) remains classified as mixed epithelial and mesenchymal tumors in the updated WHO classification 4th edition; however, it is still regarded as a subset of endometrial carcinoma based on its pattern of spread and the fact that mutation profiles resemble endometrial serous and endometrioid carcinomas [26–28]. Sarcomatous transdifferentiation of the underlying endometrial carcinoma has been hypothesized [29–31], and CS is now considered and treated as a high-grade epithelial tumor [32]. Therefore, CS should not be categorized as uterine sarcomas.

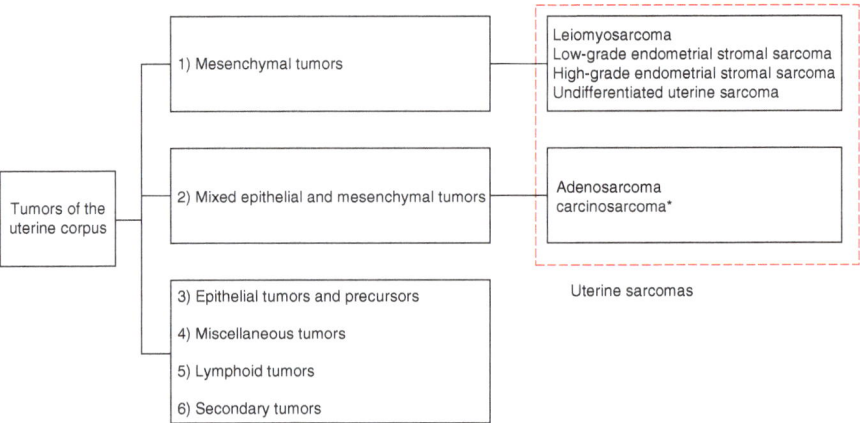

Fig. 7.1 WHO classification of tumors of the uterine corpus and histopathological subtypes of uterine sarcomas (4th edition, 2014) [25] (*Carcinosarcoma is no longer considered a uterine sarcoma. *WHO* World Health Organization)

LMS is a malignant smooth-muscle tumor and is the most common type of US with an incidence of 63% [27, 33]. Epithelioid and myxoid LMS are two histopathological variants that differ from the ordinary spindle cell leiomyosarcoma [25]. LMS has a poor prognosis even in tumors confined to the uterus with only a slightly better 5-year survival in myxoid LMS (73%), compared to ordinary LMS (49%) [27, 34]. LMS at stage II has a 5-year survival of 25%, with no patients alive at 5 years when tumor spreads outside the pelvis [34]. Recurrence rates are from 53% to 71% [2, 35].

Endometrial stromal sarcomas (ESS) are the second most common mesenchymal tumor of the uterus (21%) and resemble the endometrial stroma in the proliferative phase [25, 33]. Currently, molecular studies have identified genetic signatures that support a subdivision of ESS into low- and high-grade entities, despite no typical histopathological features in this classification [36]. New evidence support that JAZF1-SUZ12 (formerly JAZF1-JJAZ1) gene fusion caused by t(7;17)(p15;q21) translocation is present in low-grade ESS (LG-ESS) [15, 37–39], while YWHAE-FAM22A/B translocation defines high-grade ESS (HG-ESS) [36]. Patients with LG-ESS and FIGO stages I and II have a 5-year survival rate greater than 90%, while patients with advanced stages of the disease have significantly lower rates between 40% and 50% [15, 40]. Recurrence in LG-ESS is common and greater in advanced stage disease. Patients with HG-ESS usually present with advanced stage disease, and progression is more common compared with LG-ESS. Mean OS is between 1 and 2 years [1]. At present, molecular analyses are not used in routine pathologic evaluation, but are helpful to classify difficult cases and are potential future therapeutic targets.

Undifferentiated uterine sarcoma (UUS) arises in the endometrium or myometrium with high-grade cytological features and no specific type of differentiation [25]. UUS lacks resemblance to the proliferative phase of endometrial stroma and exhibits a complex karyotype with no specific translocation [36]. It is a rare tumor, and the diagnosis is one of exclusions of the more commonly encountered differentiated US, such as LMS and AS [36]. When patients are diagnosed with this aggressive tumor, it is usually in the advanced stage (>60%) and has worse survival when compared with LG/HG-ESS. Five-year survival is <50%, and even patients with stage I tumors die within 2 years [25].

Adenosarcoma (AS) is a mixed tumor in which the epithelial component is benign or atypical and the stromal component is low-grade malignant [25].The stromal component usually are low grade (approximately 90% of cases), but when at least 25% of the tumor corresponds with high grade, it is classified as an AS with sarcomatous overgrowth (ASSO). AS represents 5–10% of all US and ASSO is seen in 8–54% of AS [41, 42]. Recurrences are usually composed exclusively of mesenchymal elements and occur in 15–25% of AS or 45–70% of ASSO [1, 27]. Five-year survival for patients with AS in early-stage disease is 79% decreasing to 48% in patients with stage III disease. Mortality in patients with AS is 10–25% while in patients with ASSO can rise to 75%. Thus, patients with tumors exhibiting sarcomatous overgrowth have the poorest outcomes [1].

7.3   Clinical Presentation of Peritoneal Sarcomatosis

The mean age of presentation for US is 50 years, but it may arise at any age. Clinicians may encounter PS that has developed several years after hysterectomy or uterine surgeries for benign conditions. Frequently, retrospective reevaluation of pathology reports reveals sarcoma. Cases of PS after laparoscopic or robotic access with morcellation or slicing of uterine fibroids have been reported [10, 11, 43]. Considering the high risk of occult US in women over 50 years, caution should be used when minimally invasive surgery is performed [44]. Currently this treatment modality is under moratorium.

Patients usually experience symptoms that are nonspecific and that vary in intensity secondary to pelvic involvement. As patients become symptomatic, it is due to either tumor invasion into the adjacent organs (urinary, rectal, or vascular symptoms) or mass effect in the peritoneal cavity, which is often described as early satiety, bloating, or unintentional weight loss [21]. The problem of late diagnosis may be explained by the fact that the tumor has a lot of space to grow before any symptoms occur.

7.4   Management

In patients where a complete resection may be feasible, the first-line treatment for US is surgery, whether the disease is limited to the uterus or with metastatic spread [45].

7.4.1   Systemic Chemotherapy

Local recurrence or metastatic disease from US is a challenging condition to treat. There are a limited number of studies that evaluate the role of the different treatment modalities available today; however, palliative surgery and systemic chemotherapy are the most commonly used treatment, which may also be the only treatment available for patients with locally advanced, recurrent, metastatic, or inoperable initial presentation of the tumor. The median OS of patients with advanced or metastatic US is less than a year, and the median PFS is only 4 months for patients treated with systemic chemotherapy and CRS [46]. In a phase III study, Reed et al. have shown that adjuvant chemotherapy in patients with LMS did not significantly improve OS [47].

The National Comprehensive Cancer Network (NCCN) guidelines recommend either a single agent or a combination of two cytotoxic agents for systemic management of US based on the consensus of acceptable approaches to treatment by gynecologic and medical oncologists [32] (Table 7.1).

Historically, PS and advanced US with metastases have had very limited response to systemic chemotherapy. Patients who received anthracyclines and ifosfamide

Table 7.1 Systemic chemotherapy for uterine sarcoma

Single-agent options	Combination regimens
Dacarbazine	Docetaxel/gemcitabine
Docetaxel	Doxorubicin/dacarbazine
Doxorubicin	Doxorubicin/ifosfamide
Epirubicin	Gemcitabine/dacarbazine
Eribulin	Gemcitabine/vinorelbine
Gemcitabine	
Ifosfamide	
Liposomal doxorubicin	
Pazopanib	
Temozolomide	
Trabectedin	
Vinorelbine	

Based on NCCN guidelines version 2. 2016

(i.e., doxorubicin/ifosfamide) had a median survival of 1 year [48]. Gemcitabine with or without docetaxel has been used for palliative treatment. Demetri et al. demonstrated the effectiveness of trabectedin in patients with advanced LMS, with median OS of 12 months in patients with metastatic LMS [49].

Pautier et al. showed significant improvement of PFS at 3 years (55%) in patients with LMS treated with doxorubicin/ifosfamide/cisplatin and subsequent radiotherapy, although, this treatment had high toxicity rates [50]. Similar PFS (57%) with lesser toxicity was obtained in patients treated with docetaxel/gemcitabine followed by doxorubicin. This combination also has the highest response rate with median OS of 16 months as a first-line option in patients with metastatic US and 15 months as a second-line modality [20, 51, 52].

Different chemotherapeutic agents have been studied in order to find a monotherapeutic regimens or combinations of drugs for systemic chemotherapy in patients with advanced US. Complete response (CR) varied between 2% and 9% and partial response (PR) in the range of 13–44%. CR+PR have been found in 10–53% patients with OS and PFS between 12–26 months and 4–7 months, respectively (Table 7.2).

Eribulin, a microtubule binder which inhibits mitotic activity, shows better results than trabectedin as a single-agent modality in LMS patients with median OS of 14 months, while dacarbazine has had a significantly lower median OS of 12, ($p < 0.05$) [57]. Trabectedin was not included by the NCCN, since it was only approved in October 2015 as therapy for LMS.

Hormonal treatment has been used in combination with chemotherapy and might be beneficial in some patients. US may express estrogen and progesterone receptors (ER/PR) and, therefore, a target for hormonal therapy with drugs such as medroxyprogesterone acetate, megestrol, aromatase inhibitors, and gonadotropin-releasing hormone (GnRH) analogs [58]. Clinicians should bear in mind that the percentage of ER/PR positive tumors may vary among different histopathological types. It has been shown that among stromal sarcomas, 83% of LG-ESS express ER/PR, while

Table 7.2 Chemotherapy agents in metastatic uterine sarcoma with response rates and overall survival

Author	Chemotherapy agent	No. for analysis	CR	PR	CR+PR rate (95% confidence interval)	Median OS time (mos)	Median PFS (mos)
Hensley et al. [19]	Gemcitabine/ docetaxel	34	9%	44%	53% (35–70)	17.9	5.6 (4.3–9.9)
Hensley et al. [20]	Gemcitabine/ docetaxel (1st line)	42	5%	31%	36%	16.1 (4–41.3)	4.4 (0.4–37)
Hensley et al. [51]	Gemcitabine/ docetaxel (2st line)	48	6%	21%	27%	14.7 (0.8–50.9)	6.7 (0.7–27)
Omura et al. [53]	Doxorubicin	28	NR	NR	25% (9–41)	12.1	NR
Look et al. [54]	Gemcitabine	42	2%	19%	21% (7–31)	NR	NR
Sutton et al. [55]	Liposomal doxorubicin	32	3%	13%	16%	NR	NR
Monk et al. [56]	Trabectedin	20	NR	10%	10%	26.1	5.8

CR complete response, *mos* months, *NR* not reported, *OS* overall survival, *PFS* progression-free survival, *PR* partial response

only 10% of USS with nuclear uniformity express ER/PR [59]. ER/PR expression may be completely absent in USS with nuclear polymorphism, while LMS expression ranges between 30% and 80% [60, 61]. Patients with ER-negative sarcomas have demonstrated poor OS (median OS of 16 months) when compared to ER-positive sarcomas (median OS of 36 months), with ER positivity being an independent predictor of improved OS [6, 58].

7.4.2 Radiotherapy

Various authors reported controversial results regarding radiotherapy in patients with US. Although radiotherapy has shown some efficacy in patients with uterine carcinosarcoma, there is no significant improvement of OS in patients after adjuvant radiotherapy in ESS, since tumor relapse of the tumor is predominantly distant [62]. In addition, LMS histopathological subtype does not respond well to this treatment modality [47]. Additionally, radiotherapy did not improve local or distant recurrence rates; however, local pelvic radiation and brachytherapy may be beneficial in patients with cervical stromal involvement [63]. Meanwhile, Weitmann et al. have shown that radiotherapy in combination with surgical treatment may improve the OS (81% in 5 years) and provide local control in patients with ESS histopathological subtype of US [63].

While the overall role of radiotherapy is very limited, it may be useful in case of symptomatic recurrence or metastasis as a palliative treatment, when other treatment modalities are not feasible or may not improve patient quality of life [63].

7.4.3 Palliative Surgery

US with PS has a wide variety of clinical presentations. As with most malignancies, prognosis is better when detected early. Even with an aggressive surgical approach, including tumor debulking with negative margins and systemic chemotherapy, recurrence with locally advanced tumor may occur. These patients are the most difficult to manage, and often, the only treatment modality is a palliative approach [21].

The goal of palliative management is to alleviate symptoms, which in turn may improve the quality of life in suffering patients. Surgery is performed without curative intent; however, even palliative debulking of tumor may prolong life and improve quality of life. Additionally, surgery in incurable patients, may prevent development of bowel obstruction, respiratory difficulty, or ureteral and vena cava compression syndromes [21].

Patients with advanced, incurable malignancy should be considered candidates for palliative surgical treatment if resection, with or without radiation therapy, can be carried out with limited morbidity. Even partial resection of tumor with retroperitoneal extension can improve symptoms in up to 75% of patients [64].

7.4.4 CRS/HIPEC in Patients with PS from US

7.4.4.1 Introduction

Systemic chemotherapy, radiation therapy, and surgery have had minimal success in the management of patients with PS from US. Median OS using these modalities is between 15 and 29 months, supporting the necessity to develop new therapeutic approaches.

Patients with peritoneal disease from gastrointestinal or gynecological epithelial cancers (peritoneal carcinomatosis) have demonstrated improved outcomes following cytoreductive surgery combined with hyperthermic intraperitoneal chemotherapy [65–75]. The rational of this dual approach is based on the assumption that surgery alone may not provide adequate local disease control; therefore, a complete cytoreduction, to remove all gross disease and reduce it to microscopic levels, coupled with delivery of hyperthermic intraperitoneal chemotherapy to eradicate microscopic tumor cells is required [76].

7.4.5   Previous Studies

The literature on CRS/HIPEC in patients with PS from US is limited. Several studies have evaluated this modality in patients with PS, but, due to the rarity of the disease, most studies consist of a combination of histopathological types. This tumor heterogeneity should be kept in mind, since tumor aggressiveness and biological behavior differ and will introduce bias when the overall outcomes are analyzed (Table 7.3).

One of the first studies that used CRS/HIPEC in patients with PS was carried out by Berthet et al. [77], who studied 43 patients with recurrent abdominopelvic sarcoma from different origins between 1989 and 1996. The histological subtypes varied with just four patients with tumors arising from the uterus. Intraperitoneal chemotherapy was performed in 30 patients with complete cytoreduction: 16 HIPEC with cisplatin/doxorubicin ($n = 3$) or cisplatin followed by early postoperative intraperitoneal chemotherapy (EPIC) with doxorubicin ($n = 13$) and 14 EPIC with cisplatin/doxorubicin ($n = 7$) or doxorubicin ($n = 7$) alone. The remaining 13 patients were managed with cytoreductive surgery ($n = 13$) without any chemotherapy. The median survival was 20 months for all patients. Those with a complete cytoreduction plus intraperitoneal chemotherapy demonstrated an improved 5-year survival when compared to patients who received surgery alone (39% versus 0%, respectively).

Eilber et al. [78] published another prospective study in 54 patients with recurrent abdominal sarcoma enrolled between 1990 and 1997. Fourteen patients had primary US. Patients were divided by stage II ($n = 35$) or stage III ($n = 19$) according to the presence of hepatic metastases at the time of presentation. All patients underwent CRS/EPIC with mitoxantrone (20 mg/m^2). Forty-five patients (83%) recurred with a mean interval to recurrence of 11 months (median, 9 months, and range, 1–53 months). Peritoneal and liver recurrence rates were 48% and 69%, respectively. Overall 5-year survival was 31%, with the best results in the stage II group compared with the stage III group, 46% and 5%, respectively. Although the study did not describe how many patients with primary US were included in each group, they concluded that CRS/EPIC with mitoxantrone significantly lowered the rate of peritoneal recurrence and provides benefit for patients with disease limited to the peritoneum.

Between 1997 and 2002, Rossi et al. [23] conducted a multicenter prospective study in 60 patients with a diagnosis of advanced (multifocal primary or local recurrent disease), intra-abdominal visceral or retroperitoneal soft tissue sarcoma who underwent adequate cytoreductive surgery (tumor remnants <3 mm in greatest

Table 7.3 Clinical outcomes of CRS/HIPEC for peritoneal sarcomatosis from uterine sarcoma

Author/publication date (ref)	N	US n (%)	Histopathological subtypes	Clinical presentation	Treatment modalities and HIPEC/EPIC chemotherapy	CC 0–1 n (%)	Recurrence n (%)	Median OS (mos)	5-year survival	Morbidity/mortality n (%)
Berthet et al./1999 [77]	43	4 (9)	LMS (22), LPS (9), FBS (4), SRCS (4), SCC (2), Schw (1), HPC (1)	Recurrent (43)	-CRS/HIPEC: CDDP/DOX (3) -CRS/HIPEC + EPIC: CDDP + DOX (13) –CRS + EPIC: CDDP/DOX (7) or DOX (7) – CRS (13)	27 (63)	NR	20	30% CRS/HIPEC or EPIC: 39% CRS alone: 0%	8 (19)/3 (7)
Eilber et al./1999 [78]	54	14 (26)	US [LMS:14], GIST (33), LPS (4), SCS (1), HS (1), OsS (1)	Recurrent (54)	-CRS/EPIC (No HIPEC): DHAD	54 (100)	8 (15) peritoneal 18 (33) peritoneal and liver 19 (35) liver	NR	31%[a] Stage I: 46% Stage II: 5%	5 (9)/0 (0)
Rossi et al./2004 [23]	60	12 (20)	US [LMS:8, ESS:4], GIST (14), RPS [LPS:20, MFH:6, Schw:4, FBS:2, SRCS:2]	Primary (29) Recurrent (31)	-CRS/HIPEC: CDDP/DOX	60 (100)[b]	27 (45) peritoneal 15 (25) peritoneal and distant	34	NR	20 (33)/0 (0)
Kusamura et al./2004 [22]	10	10 (100)	US [LMS:8, ESS:1, AS:1]	Primary (2) Recurrent (8)	-CRS/HIPEC: CDDP/MMC (2) CDDP/DOX (8)	9 (90)	3 (30) peritoneal 3 (30) peritoneal and distant	NR	65%	0 (0)/0 (0)

(continued)

Table 7.3 (continued)

Author/publication date (ref)	N	US n (%)	Histopathological subtypes	Clinical presentation	Treatment modalities and HIPEC/EPIC chemotherapy	CC 0–1 n (%)	Recurrence n (%)	Median OS (mos)	5-year survival	Morbidity/ mortality n (%)
Baratti et al./2010 [13]	37	11 (30)	US [LMS: 10, ESS: 1], RPLS (13), GIST (8), OSTS [SRCS: 3, MFS: 1, LMS: 1]	Primary (10) Recurrent (27)	-CRS/HIPEC: CDDP/DOX CDDP/MMC	31 (84)	16 (43) peritoneal 5 (14) distant	26	24%	8 (22)/1 (3)
Sugarbaker et al./2016 [11]	6	6 (100)	US [LMS: 6]	Recurrent (6)	-CRS/HIPEC/ EPIC: HIPEC: CDDP/DOX + IFO (IV) (6) EPIC: PTX (5)	6 (100)	3 (50) distant	NR	NR	2 (33)/0 (0)
Sardi et al./ Unpublished[c]	7	7 (100)	US [LMS:4, AS:2, ESS:1]	Primary (1) Recurrent (6)	-CRS/HIPEC: CDDP/DOX L-PAM	7 (100)	3 (43) peritoneal 1 (14) distant	Not reached	57%	0 (0)/0 (0)

AS adenosarcoma, CC completeness of cytoreduction score, CDDP cisplatin, CRS cytoreductive surgery, DHAD mitoxantrone, DOX doxorubicin, EPIC early postoperative intraperitoneal chemotherapy, ESS endometrial stromal sarcoma, FBS fibrosarcoma, GIST gastrointestinal stromal sarcoma, HIPEC hyperthermic intraperitoneal chemotherapy, HPC hemangiopericytoma, HS hemangiosarcoma, IFO ifosfamide, IV intravenous, LMS leiomyosarcoma, L-PAM melphalan, LPS liposarcoma, MFH malignant fibrous histiocytoma, MFS myxofibrosarcoma, MMC mitomycin-C, mos months, NR not reported, OS overall survival, OsS osteosarcoma, OSTS other soft tissue sarcoma, PTX paclitaxel, RPLP retroperitoneal liposarcoma, RPS retroperitoneal sarcoma, SCC spindle cell carcinoma, Schw schwannoma, SCS synovial cell sarcoma, SRCS small round cell sarcoma, US uterine sarcoma
[a]Stage I or II according to hepatic metastases at presentation
[b]Patients received complete cytoreduction (68%) or near-complete cytoreduction (tumor residual <3 mm) (32%)
[c]Presented in 9th International Congress on Peritoneal Surface Malignancies, Amsterdam, Netherlands, 2014

dimensions) and HIPEC with doxorubicin (15.25 mg/L) and cisplatin (43 mg/L). Twelve of those patients (20%) had sarcomatosis arising from US, eight LMS and four ESS. The median overall survival and median time to local disease progression in all patients was 34 months and 22 months, respectively. No separate data for patients with PS from US was presented. There were no postoperative deaths and morbidity rate was 33%. They found that the extent of cytoreduction (no macroscopic evident tumor vs. tumor residuals <3 mm in greatest dimension) influences overall and local progression-free survival, supporting the pivotal role of surgery to control disease. It was also stated that the antineoplastic activity of HIPEC might be clouded by the intrinsic differences in the drug sensitivity of each tumor due to the heterogeneity of the histological types included. Their findings were encouraging, suggesting improved local control but with substantial toxicity and the need to further explore this approach due to the absence of effective systemic agents.

Kusamura et al. [22] reported the first homogeneous series of US treated by CRS/HIPEC. In their study, ten patients with primary ($n = 2$) or recurrent ($n = 8$) US treated with CRS/HIPEC were enrolled from 1997 to 2001. In nine cases complete cytoreduction (CC 0–1) was achieved, and HIPEC was performed with cisplatin/ doxorubicin ($n = 8$) or cisplatin/mitomycin-C ($n = 2$). No surgical complications, toxicity, or perioperative mortality occurred. Six patients recurred with a median PFS of 15 months after a median follow-up of 25 months (2–61 months). Five-year OS of 65% and 5-year PFS of 30% were encouraging, compared to historical controls presenting with OS rates from 0% to 20% in advanced stages, suggesting that CRS/HIPEC might offer the best results in patients with PS from US. These findings warrant further investigation.

Baratti et al. [13] performed a prospective database review of 37 patients who underwent CRS/HIPEC with cisplatin (45 ml/l) plus doxorubicin (15 mg/l) or cisplatin (25 ml/m²/l) plus mitomycin-C (3.3 mg/m²/l) from 1996 to 2006 at the National Cancer Institute in Milan, Italy. Eleven patients (30%) had sarcomatosis arising from US; eight represented recurrences with 73% high-grade tumors. Thirty-one patients underwent a complete CRS (CC-0 and CC-1) of which ten had sarcomatosis from US. More than 20% of the patients presented with grade 3–4 complications, and 1 surgical mortality was reported in a patient in the US group. In all patients, the median OS was 26 months (5-year OS of 24.3%) with seven patients demonstrating a survival over 40 months. The median locoregional progression-free survival (LRPFS) was 12 months, and the median distant progression-free survival (DPFS) was 80 months. Sarcomatosis from uterine LMS had the best median LRPFS and greater median OS rates (15 months and 30 months, respectively). Use of mitomycin-C and residual disease after CRS was correlated with low LRPFS and DPFS. Five of 11 patients with US were alive 4–10 years after CRS-HIPEC. This study highlighted the impact of a complete cytoreduction for patients with low-grade PS, with encouraging long-term results in patients with disseminated uterine LMS, which warrant further clinical investigations.

In 2016, Sugarbaker et al. reported six patients with PS after morcellation of uterine LMS who underwent CRS/HIPEC with cisplatin (50 mg/m²)/doxorubicin (15 mg/m²) with the addition of continuous intravenous infusion of ifosfamide

(1300 mg/m^2) during the 90 min HIPEC procedure. Patients then received EPIC with paclitaxel (20 mg/m^2) on postoperative days 1 through 5. There was no associated mortality and grade III/IV complications occurred in two patients. Three patients recurred and one later died. They concluded that morcellation is currently under debate, and patients with risk of sarcomatosis after laparoscopic resection or morcellation should be referred for sarcomatosis prophylaxis using the therapy they described.

At our institution, a retrospective review of a prospective database of 647 patients who underwent CRS/HIPEC showed 7 patients with PS from US between 2001 and 2014. Histopathological subtypes included LMS ($n = 4$), ASSO ($n = 2$), and ESS ($n = 1$). Complete cytoreduction was achieved in all patients and HIPEC was performed with melphalan (50 mg/m^2) in six patients with recurrent disease and with doxorubicin (7 mg/m^2) plus cisplatin (50 mg/m^2) in one patient with primary malignancy. There were no grades III/IV complications or hospital mortality. Three patients recurred in the peritoneum and one patient in the liver. Two of three patients with recurrence died, and one underwent multiple procedures and is currently without evidence of disease 28 months after the first CRS/HIPEC. One patient with extraperitoneal metastatic disease underwent multiple procedures that included liver resection, wedge resection of lung, and a left ductal mastectomy. The patient has no evidence of disease 172 months after CRS/HIPEC and is 54 months out from resection of metastases. Five-year OS was 57% and 3-year PFS of 38% with a median PFS of 20 months. There are currently five patients with no evidence of disease with a median follow-up of 37 months (range 18–172 months). We found that among carefully selected patients, CRS/HIPEC can be safely performed in specialized centers and is a feasible treatment modality for PS from US, with complete cytoreduction, low morbidity, and promising survival.

A multi-institutional retrospective review is currently underway of patient data with PS from US treated with CRS/HIPEC to better understand the role of HIPEC in the management of this disease. Seven specialized centers around the world (Baltimore, MD USA; Washington DC, USA; Chicago, IL USA; Milan, Italy; Rome, Italy; Lyon, France and Osaka, Japan) are participating in the study. Thirty-six patients have undergone 38 CRS/HIPEC procedures from 2005 to 2014. Histopathology includes LMS, USS, LG-ESS, and AS in 17, 12, 3, and 3 patients, respectively. HIPEC was performed with cisplatin/doxorubicin ($n = 22$), cisplatin/mitomycin ($n = 2$), melphalan ($n = 10$), mitomycin-C ($n = 2$), cisplatin ($n = 1$), and unknown in one case. Complete cytoreduction was achieved in 34 procedures (90%), and five patients (14%) experienced grade III–V complications. Two surgery-related deaths occurred on postoperative days 26 and 88. Fifty-six percent of patients with complete cytoreduction recurred: 16 in peritoneum, 8 chest, 3 retroperitoneum, 2 liver, 1 bone, 1 vaginal stump, and 1 abdominal wall with 4 patients (11%) presenting with multiple sites of recurrence. Adjuvant chemotherapy was gemcitabine/docetaxel ($n = 5$), doxorubicin/ifosfamide ($n = 5$), and EPIC with paclitaxel ($n = 5$). OS at 1, 3, and 5 years was 75%, 53%, and 32%, respectively, with median OS of 37 months. PFS was calculated in 32 patients with complete cytoreduction and sufficient available data. The 1-, 3-, and 5-year PFS was 67%, 32%, and 32%, respectively, with median PFS of 19 months. CRS/HIPEC appears to be a promising treatment modality for patients with PS with a goal of complete cytoreduction similar across international centers. Unfortunately, there is a significant discordance in selecting regional and systemic chemotherapy, and a global prospective registry of patients is needed to further assess the efficacy of CRS/HIPEC.

7.4.6 Surgical Approach and Technical Considerations

The surgical approach of CRS/HIPEC has been well described by Sugarbaker [76] and others [79]. However, there are different characteristics in the presentation and the technical approaches needed for CRS/HIPEC in patients with PS from US when compared to peritoneal carcinomatosis from other malignancies.

1. Rapid tumor growth may occur within the first few weeks or months following initial surgery and may result in patients presenting with large symptomatic masses and subsequently not being considered for surgery (Fig. 7.2).
2. These tumors frequently have less involvement in the upper abdomen and are less infiltrative into the bowel; thus, extensive bowel resections are less common.
3. The majority of these patients have had prior extensive and, often, multiple pelvic surgeries and wide-field radiation, therefore, making further resections difficult due to the degree of pelvic involvement. Consequently, surgery is complex due to peritoneal adhesions, tumor recurrence in scar tissue, and distortion of normal anatomy, resulting in prolonged surgical time. Furthermore, extensive pelvic peritonectomies with iliac vessel and ureter resections are common and the most challenging components of the surgery. These resections are generally not necessary in peritoneal carcinomatosis from other malignancies.
4. The selection of intraperitoneal chemotherapy agents is a major consideration, especially in recurrent disease. Traditionally, cisplatin and doxorubicin have been used in the treatment of PS in patients undergoing CRS/HIPEC; however, sarcomas are generally considered chemoresistant tumors. Melphalan has been used for recurrent tumors of the gastrointestinal and gynecologic tracts with good results [80].

   Melphalan has been described as a successful agent in the treatment of aggressive chemoresistant neoplasms, such as soft tissue sarcomas and melanomas of the extremities [81, 82]. Alkylating agents such as melphalan, cyclophosphamide, and ifosfamide have the highest activation energy by hyperthermia [83, 84], with melphalan having the greatest thermal cytotoxic enhancement and drug penetration into the tumor [85, 86]. Melphalan is also the primary drug of choice for primary PS at our institution, although no comparable studies are available.

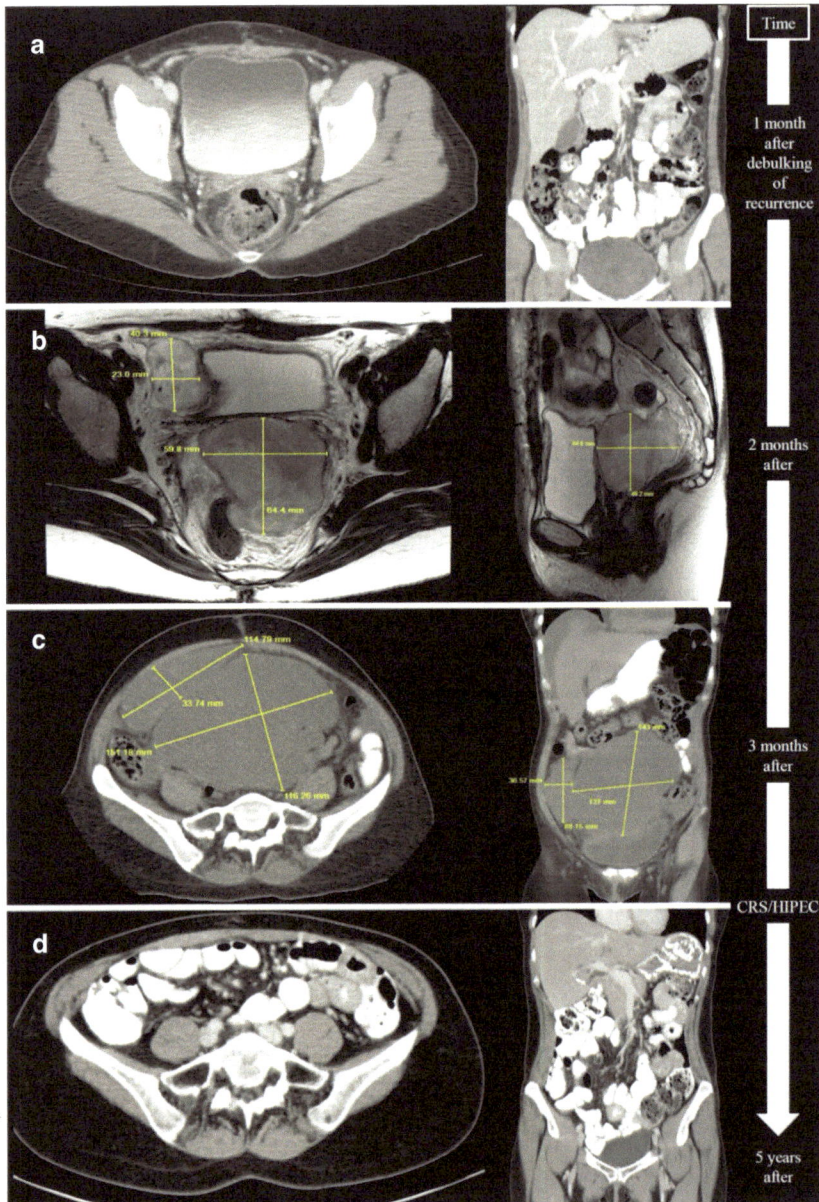

Fig. 7.2 Rapid tumor growth in a patient with peritoneal sarcomatosis from uterine leiomyosarcoma. (**a**) Computed tomography (CT) scan 1 month after debulking of pelvic recurrence; no evidence of disease. (**b**) Magnetic resonance imaging of the pelvis 2 months after the abovementioned debulking showing two pelvic masses (6×6×5 cm and 2×4×5 cm). (**c**) Abdominopelvic CT scan 1 day before CRS/HIPEC and 3 months after debulking of recurrence showing rapidly growing tumors (15×11×14 cm and 3×11×9 cm). (**d**) CT scan 5 years after CRS/HIPEC showing no evidence of disease recurrence. *CRS/HIPEC* cytoreductive surgery and hyperthermic intraperitoneal chemotherapy

7.5 Conclusion

Peritoneal sarcomatosis from uterine sarcoma seems to have better outcomes with CRS/HIPEC when compared to peritoneal sarcomatosis of other origins.

Complete cytoreduction is the cornerstone in the management of these patients and the most important factor to improve overall and progression-free survival.

Hyperthermic intraperitoneal chemotherapy plays a role in the control of peritoneal recurrence and provides benefit for patients with disease limited to the peritoneum. This can be performed with acceptable morbidity and mortality when compared to historical controls.

The heterogeneity in histological types and intrinsic differences in the drug sensitivity of each tumor are important variables when evaluating HIPEC. Further prospective studies are needed.

References

1. Denschlag D, Thiel FC, Ackermann S, et al. Sarcoma of the uterus. Guideline of the DGGG (S2k-Level, AWMF Registry No. 015/074, August 2015). Geburtshilfe Frauenheilkd. 2015;75(10):1028–42.
2. Major FJ, Blessing JA, Silverberg SG, et al. Prognostic factors in early-stage uterine sarcoma. A Gynecologic Oncology Group study. Cancer. 1993;71(4 Suppl):1702–9.
3. Siegel RL, Miller KD, Jemal A. Cancer statistics, 2016. CA Cancer J Clin. 2016;66(1):7–30.
4. Brooks SE, Zhan M, Cote T, Baquet CR. Surveillance, epidemiology, and end results analysis of 2677 cases of uterine sarcoma 1989-1999. Gynecol Oncol. 2004;93(1):204–8.
5. Sherman ME, Devesa SS. Analysis of racial differences in incidence, survival, and mortality for malignant tumors of the uterine corpus. Cancer. 2003;98(1):176–86.
6. Thanopoulou E, Aleksic A, Thway K, Khabra K, Judson I. Hormonal treatments in metastatic endometrial stromal sarcomas: the 10-year experience of the sarcoma unit of Royal Marsden Hospital. Clin Sarcoma Res. 2015;5:8.
7. Samuji M, O'Sullivan R, Shireen R. Uterine sarcoma after tamoxifen therapy for breast cancer. Ir Med J. 2013;106(8):246.
8. Launonen V, Vierimaa O, Kiuru M, et al. Inherited susceptibility to uterine leiomyomas and renal cell cancer. Proc Natl Acad Sci U S A. 2001;98(6):3387–92.
9. Yu CL, Tucker MA, Abramson DH, et al. Cause-specific mortality in long-term survivors of retinoblastoma. J Natl Cancer Inst. 2009;101(8):581–91.
10. Kho KA, Lin K, Hechanova M, Richardson DL. Risk of occult uterine sarcoma in women undergoing hysterectomy for benign indications. Obstet Gynecol. 2016;127(3):468–73.
11. Sugarbaker P, Ihemelandu C, Bijelic L. Cytoreductive surgery and HIPEC as a treatment option for laparoscopic resection of uterine leiomyosarcoma with morcellation: early results. Ann Surg Oncol. 2016;23(5):1501–7.
12. Jimenez WA, Sardi A, Nieroda C, Gushchin V. Cytoreductive surgery and hyperthermic intraperitoneal chemotherapy in the management of recurrent high-grade uterine sarcoma with peritoneal dissemination. Am J Obstet Gynecol. 2014;210(3):259. e251–258
13. Baratti D, Pennacchioli E, Kusamura S, et al. Peritoneal sarcomatosis: is there a subset of patients who may benefit from cytoreductive surgery and hyperthermic intraperitoneal chemotherapy? Ann Surg Oncol. 2010;17(12):3220–8.
14. Gadducci A, Sartori E, Landoni F, et al. The prognostic relevance of histological type in uterine sarcomas: a Cooperation Task Force (CTF) multivariate analysis of 249 cases. Eur J Gynaecol Oncol. 2002;23(4):295–9.

15. Leath 3rd CA, Huh WK, Hyde Jr J, et al. A multi-institutional review of outcomes of endometrial stromal sarcoma. Gynecol Oncol. 2007;105(3):630–4.
16. Inoue D, Yamamoto M, Sugita G, Kurokawa T, Yoshida Y. Debulking surgery and hyperthermic intraperitoneal chemotherapy in the management of a recurrent aggressive uterine myxoid leiomyosarcoma with peritoneal dissemination. Gynecol Oncol Rep. 2015;13:60–3.
17. Karakousis CP, Blumenson LE, Canavese G, Rao U. Surgery for disseminated abdominal sarcoma. Am J Surg. 1992;163(6):560–4.
18. Bonvalot S, Cavalcanti A, Le Pechoux C, et al. Randomized trial of cytoreduction followed by intraperitoneal chemotherapy versus cytoreduction alone in patients with peritoneal sarcomatosis. Eur J Surg Oncol. 2005;31(8):917–23.
19. Hensley ML, Maki R, Venkatraman E, et al. Gemcitabine and docetaxel in patients with unresectable leiomyosarcoma: results of a phase II trial. J Clin Oncol. 2002;20(12):2824–31.
20. Hensley ML, Blessing JA, Mannel R, Rose PG. Fixed-dose rate gemcitabine plus docetaxel as first-line therapy for metastatic uterine leiomyosarcoma: a Gynecologic Oncology Group phase II trial. Gynecol Oncol. 2008;109(3):329–34.
21. Sheldon DG, James TA, Kraybill WG. Palliative surgery of soft tissue sarcoma. Surg Oncol Clin N Am. 2004;13(3):531–41. ix
22. Kusamura S, Raspagliesi F, Baratti D, Gronchi A, Casali P, Deraco M. Uterine sarcoma treated by cytoreductive surgery and intraperitoneal hyperthermic perfusion: a feasibility study. J Chemother. 2004;16(Suppl 5):19–22.
23. Rossi CR, Deraco M, De Simone M, et al. Hyperthermic intraperitoneal intraoperative chemotherapy after cytoreductive surgery for the treatment of abdominal sarcomatosis: clinical outcome and prognostic factors in 60 consecutive patients. Cancer. 2004;100(9):1943–50.
24. Abu-Zaid A, Azzam A, Abuzaid M, et al. Cytoreductive surgery plus hyperthermic intraperitoneal chemotherapy for management of peritoneal sarcomatosis: a preliminary single-center experience from Saudi Arabia. Gastroenterol Res Pract. 2016;2016:6567473.
25. Kurman RJ, Carcangiu ML, Herrington CS, Young RH. WHO classification of tumours. WHO classification of tumours of female reproductive organs, vol. 6. Lyon-Paris. WHO Press; 2014, p. 307.
26. McConechy MK, Ding J, Cheang MC, et al. Use of mutation profiles to refine the classification of endometrial carcinomas. J Pathol. 2012;228(1):20–30.
27. Prat J, Mbatani. Uterine sarcomas. Int J Gynaecol Obstet. 2015;131(Suppl 2):S105–10.
28. McConechy MK, Hoang LN, Chui MH, et al. In-depth molecular profiling of the biphasic components of uterine carcinosarcomas. J Pathol Clin Res. 2015;1(3):173–85.
29. Watanabe M, Shimizu K, Kato H, et al. Carcinosarcoma of the uterus: immunohistochemical and genetic analysis of clonality of one case. Gynecol Oncol. 2001;82(3):563–7.
30. Jin Z, Ogata S, Tamura G, et al. Carcinosarcomas (malignant mullerian mixed tumors) of the uterus and ovary: a genetic study with special reference to histogenesis. Int J Gynecol Pathol. 2003;22(4):368–73.
31. Kernochan LE, Garcia RL. Carcinosarcomas (malignant mixed Mullerian tumor) of the uterus: advances in elucidation of biologic and clinical characteristics. J Natl Compr Cancer Netw. 2009;7(5):550–6. quiz 557
32. Network. NCC. Uterine neoplasms (Version 2.2016). https://www.nccn.org/professionals/physician_gls/pdf/uterine.pdf. Accessed 21 Jul 2016.
33. Trope CG, Abeler VM, Kristensen GB. Diagnosis and treatment of sarcoma of the uteru. A review. Acta Oncol. 2012;51(6):694–705.
34. Abeler VM, Royne O, Thoresen S, Danielsen HE, Nesland JM, Kristensen GB. Uterine sarcomas in Norway. A histopathological and prognostic survey of a total population from 1970 to 2000 including 419 patients. Histopathology. 2009;54(3):355–64.
35. Koivisto-Korander R, Butzow R, Koivisto AM, Leminen A. Clinical outcome and prognostic factors in 100 cases of uterine sarcoma: experience in Helsinki University Central Hospital 1990–2001. Gynecol Oncol. 2008;111(1):74–81.

36. Conklin CM, Longacre TA. Endometrial stromal tumors: the new WHO classification. Adv Anat Pathol. 2014;21(6):383–93.
37. Lee CH, Marino-Enriquez A, Ou W, et al. The clinicopathologic features of YWHAE-FAM22 endometrial stromal sarcomas: a histologically high-grade and clinically aggressive tumor. Am J Surg Pathol. 2012;36(5):641–53.
38. Lax SF. Molecular genetic changes in epithelial, stromal and mixed neoplasms of the endometrium. Pathology. 2007;39(1):46–54.
39. Huang HY, Ladanyi M, Soslow RA. Molecular detection of JAZF1-JJAZ1 gene fusion in endometrial stromal neoplasms with classic and variant histology: evidence for genetic heterogeneity. Am J Surg Pathol. 2004;28(2):224–32.
40. Chang KL, Crabtree GS, Lim-Tan SK, Kempson RL, Hendrickson MR. Primary uterine endometrial neoplasms. A clinicopathologic study of 117 cases. Am J Surg Pathol. 1990;14(5):415–38.
41. Clement PB, Scully RE. Mullerian adenosarcoma of the uterus: a clinicopathologic analysis of 100 cases with a review of the literature. Hum Pathol. 1990;21(4):363–81.
42. Gallardo A, Prat J. Mullerian adenosarcoma: a clinicopathologic and immunohistochemical study of 55 cases challenging the existence of adenofibroma. Am J Surg Pathol. 2009;33(2):278–88.
43. Bogani G, Chiappa V, Ditto A, et al. Morcellation of undiagnosed uterine sarcoma: a critical review. Crit Rev Oncol Hematol. 2016;98:302–8.
44. Rodriguez AM, Asoglu MR, Sak ME, Tan A, Borahay MA, Kilic GS. Incidence of occult leiomyosarcoma in presumed morcellation cases: a database study. Eur J Obstet Gynecol Reprod Biol. 2016;197:31–5.
45. Dizon DS, Birrer MJ. Advances in the diagnosis and treatment of uterine sarcomas. Discov Med. 2014;17(96):339–45.
46. Ray-Coquard I, Rizzo E, Blay JY, et al. Impact of chemotherapy in uterine sarcoma (UtS): review of 13 clinical trials from the EORTC Soft Tissue and Bone Sarcoma Group (STBSG) involving advanced/metastatic UtS compared to other soft tissue sarcoma (STS) patients treated with first line chemotherapy. Gynecol Oncol. 2016;142(1):95–101.
47. Reed NS, Mangioni C, Malmstrom H, et al. Phase III randomised study to evaluate the role of adjuvant pelvic radiotherapy in the treatment of uterine sarcomas stages I and II: an European Organisation for Research and Treatment of Cancer Gynaecological Cancer Group Study (protocol 55874). Eur J Cancer. 2008;44(6):808–18.
48. Young RJ, Natukunda A, Litiere S, Woll PJ, Wardelmann E, van der Graaf WT. First-line anthracycline-based chemotherapy for angiosarcoma and other soft tissue sarcoma subtypes: pooled analysis of eleven European Organisation for Research and Treatment of Cancer Soft Tissue and Bone Sarcoma Group trials. Eur J Cancer. 2014;50(18):3178–86.
49. Demetri GD, von Mehren M, Jones RL, et al. Efficacy and safety of trabectedin or dacarbazine for metastatic liposarcoma or leiomyosarcoma after failure of conventional chemotherapy: results of a phase III randomized multicenter clinical trial. J Clin Oncol. 2016;34(8):786–93.
50. Pautier P, Floquet A, Penel N, et al. Randomized multicenter and stratified phase II study of gemcitabine alone versus gemcitabine and docetaxel in patients with metastatic or relapsed leiomyosarcomas: a Federation Nationale des Centres de Lutte Contre le Cancer (FNCLCC) French Sarcoma Group Study (TAXOGEM study). Oncologist. 2012;17(9):1213–20.
51. Hensley ML, Blessing JA, Degeest K, Abulafia O, Rose PG, Homesley HD. Fixed-dose rate gemcitabine plus docetaxel as second-line therapy for metastatic uterine leiomyosarcoma: a Gynecologic Oncology Group phase II study. Gynecol Oncol. 2008;109(3):323–8.
52. Hensley ML, Wathen JK, Maki RG, et al. Adjuvant therapy for high-grade, uterus-limited leiomyosarcoma: results of a phase 2 trial (SARC 005). Cancer. 2013;119(8):1555–61.
53. Omura GA, Major FJ, Blessing JA, et al. A randomized study of adriamycin with and without dimethyl triazenoimidazole carboxamide in advanced uterine sarcomas. Cancer. 1983;52(4):626–32.

54. Look KY, Sandler A, Blessing JA, Lucci 3rd JA, Rose PG, Gynecologic Oncology Group S. Phase II trial of gemcitabine as second-line chemotherapy of uterine leiomyosarcoma: a Gynecologic Oncology Group (GOG) Study. Gynecol Oncol. 2004;92(2):644–7.
55. Sutton G, Blessing J, Hanjani P, Kramer P, Gynecologic Oncology G. Phase II evaluation of liposomal doxorubicin (Doxil) in recurrent or advanced leiomyosarcoma of the uterus: a Gynecologic Oncology Group study. Gynecol Oncol. 2005;96(3):749–52.
56. Monk BJ, Blessing JA, Street DG, Muller CY, Burke JJ, Hensley ML. A phase II evaluation of trabectedin in the treatment of advanced, persistent, or recurrent uterine leiomyosarcoma: a gynecologic oncology group study. Gynecol Oncol. 2012;124(1):48–52.
57. Schoffski P, Chawla S, Maki RG, et al. Eribulin versus dacarbazine in previously treated patients with advanced liposarcoma or leiomyosarcoma: a randomised, open-label, multicentre, phase 3 trial. Lancet. 2016;387(10028):1629–37.
58. Ioffe YJ, Li AJ, Walsh CS, et al. Hormone receptor expression in uterine sarcomas: prognostic and therapeutic roles. Gynecol Oncol. 2009;115(3):466–71.
59. Jakate K, Azimi F, Ali RH, et al. Endometrial sarcomas: an immunohistochemical and JAZF1 re-arrangement study in low-grade and undifferentiated tumors. Mod Pathol. 2013;26(1):95–105.
60. Leitao MM, Soslow RA, Nonaka D, et al. Tissue microarray immunohistochemical expression of estrogen, progesterone, and androgen receptors in uterine leiomyomata and leiomyosarcoma. Cancer. 2004;101(6):1455–62.
61. Kelley TW, Borden EC, Goldblum JR. Estrogen and progesterone receptor expression in uterine and extrauterine leiomyosarcomas: an immunohistochemical study. Appl Immunohistochem Mol Morphol. 2004;12(4):338–41.
62. Amant F, Floquet A, Friedlander M, et al. Gynecologic Cancer InterGroup (GCIG) consensus review for endometrial stromal sarcoma. Int J Gynecol Cancer. 2014;24(9 Suppl 3):S67–72.
63. Weitmann HD, Knocke TH, Kucera H, Potter R. Radiation therapy in the treatment of endometrial stromal sarcoma. Int J Radiat Oncol Biol Phys. 2001;49(3):739–48.
64. Shibata D, Lewis JJ, Leung DH, Brennan MF. Is there a role for incomplete resection in the management of retroperitoneal liposarcomas? J Am Coll Surg. 2001;193(4):373–9.
65. Sugarbaker PH. New standard of care for appendiceal epithelial neoplasms and pseudomyxoma peritonei syndrome? Lancet Oncol. 2006;7(1):69–76.
66. El Halabi H, Gushchin V, Francis J, et al. The role of cytoreductive surgery and heated intraperitoneal chemotherapy (CRS/HIPEC) in patients with high-grade appendiceal carcinoma and extensive peritoneal carcinomatosis. Ann Surg Oncol. 2012;19(1):110–4.
67. Lansom J, Alzahrani N, Liauw W, Morris DL. Cytoreductive surgery and hyperthermic intraperitoneal chemotherapy for pseudomyxoma peritonei and appendix tumours. Indian J Surg Oncol. 2016;7(2):166–76.
68. Jimenez W, Sardi A, Nieroda C, et al. Predictive and prognostic survival factors in peritoneal carcinomatosis from appendiceal cancer after cytoreductive surgery with hyperthermic intraperitoneal chemotherapy. Ann Surg Oncol. 2014;21(13):4218–25.
69. Sardi A, Jimenez WA, Nieroda C, Sittig M, Macdonald R, Gushchin V. Repeated cytoreductive surgery and hyperthermic intraperitoneal chemotherapy in peritoneal carcinomatosis from appendiceal cancer: analysis of survival outcomes. Eur J Surg Oncol. 2013;39(11):1207–13.
70. Yan TD, Deraco M, Baratti D, et al. Cytoreductive surgery and hyperthermic intraperitoneal chemotherapy for malignant peritoneal mesothelioma: multi-institutional experience. J Clin Oncol. 2009;27(36):6237–42.
71. Elias D, Gilly F, Boutitie F, et al. Peritoneal colorectal carcinomatosis treated with surgery and perioperative intraperitoneal chemotherapy: retrospective analysis of 523 patients from a multicentric French study. J Clin Oncol. 2010;28(1):63–8.
72. Canbay E, Yonemura Y, Brucher B, Baik SH, Sugarbaker PH. Intraperitoneal chemotherapy and its evolving role in management of gastric cancer with peritoneal metastases. Chin J Cancer Res. 2014;26(1):1–3.

73. Bijelic L, Jonson A, Sugarbaker PH. Systematic review of cytoreductive surgery and heated intraoperative intraperitoneal chemotherapy for treatment of peritoneal carcinomatosis in primary and recurrent ovarian cancer. Ann Oncol. 2007;18(12):1943–50.
74. Sun JH, Ji ZH, Yu Y, et al. Cytoreductive surgery plus hyperthermic intraperitoneal chemotherapy to treat advanced/recurrent epithelial ovarian cancer: results from a retrospective study on prospectively established database. Transl Oncol. 2016;9(2):130–8.
75. Abu-Zaid A, Azzam AZ, AlOmar O, Salem H, Amin T, Al-Badawi IA. Cytoreductive surgery and hyperthermic intraperitoneal chemotherapy for managing peritoneal carcinomatosis from endometrial carcinoma: a single-center experience of 6 cases. Ann Saudi Med. 2014;34(2):159–66.
76. Sugarbaker P. Technical handbook for the integration of cytoreductive surgery and perioperative intraperitoneal chemotherapy into the surgical management of gastrointestinal and gynecologic malignancy. 4th ed. Foundation for Applied Research in Gastrointestinal Oncology; Washington-US. 2005.
77. Berthet B, Sugarbaker TA, Chang D, Sugarbaker PH. Quantitative methodologies for selection of patients with recurrent abdominopelvic sarcoma for treatment. Eur J Cancer. 1999;35(3):413–9.
78. Eilber FC, Rosen G, Forscher C, Nelson SD, Dorey FJ, Eilber FR. Surgical resection and intraperitoneal chemotherapy for recurrent abdominal sarcomas. Ann Surg Oncol. 1999;6(7):645–50.
79. Shankar S, Ledakis P, El Halabi H, Gushchin V, Sardi A. Neoplasms of the appendix: current treatment guidelines. Hematol Oncol Clin N Am. 2012;26(6):1261–90.
80. Sardi A, Jimenez W, Nieroda C, Sittig M, Shankar S, Gushchin V. Melphalan: a promising agent in patients undergoing cytoreductive surgery and hyperthermic intraperitoneal chemotherapy. Ann Surg Oncol. 2014;21(3):908–14.
81. Jakob J, Hohenberger P. Role of isolated limb perfusion with recombinant human tumor necrosis factor alpha and melphalan in locally advanced extremity soft tissue sarcoma. Cancer. 2016;122(17):2624–32.
82. Rastrelli M, Campana LG, Valpione S, Tropea S, Zanon A, Rossi CR. Hyperthermic isolated limb perfusion in locally advanced limb soft tissue sarcoma: a 24-year single-centre experience. Int J Hyperth. 2016;32(2):165–72.
83. Urano M, Ling CC. Thermal enhancement of melphalan and oxaliplatin cytotoxicity in vitro. Int J Hyperth. 2002;18(4):307–15.
84. Takemoto M, Kuroda M, Urano M, et al. The effect of various chemotherapeutic agents given with mild hyperthermia on different types of tumours. Int J Hyperth. 2003;19(2):193–203.
85. Sugarbaker PH, Stuart OA. Pharmacokinetic and phase II study of heated intraoperative intraperitoneal melphalan. Cancer Chemother Pharmacol. 2007;59(2):151–5.
86. Mohamed F, Stuart OA, Glehen O, Urano M, Sugarbaker PH. Optimizing the factors which modify thermal enhancement of melphalan in a spontaneous murine tumor. Cancer Chemother Pharmacol. 2006;58(6):719–24.

Chapter 8
The Role of Surgery and Tyrosine Kinase Inhibitors in the Management of Advanced or Recurrent GIST

Rebecca M. Dodson, Perry Shen, Edward A. Levine, and Konstantinos I. Votanopoulos

8.1   Introduction

Gastrointestinal stromal tumors (GISTs) are the most common gastrointestinal sarcoma, accounting for 5% of all mesenchymal tumors and 1–3% of all gastrointestinal tumors. The annual incidence is 10–13 per 1,000,000, with the majority arising in the stomach (50–60%) and small bowel (20–30%) and only a minority in the large bowel (5%) and esophagus (<5%) [1, 2]. GISTs arise from activating mutations of tyrosine kinase receptors, most commonly by KIT (CD117) which is expressed in 95% of GISTs or platelet-derived growth factor receptor (PDGFR) which is mutated in 5–10% of GISTs. Yet, 10–15% have no known mutation in KIT or PDGRF and are wild type. The treatment of GISTs has dramatically changed since 2002 due to the FDA approval of imatinib/Gleevec, a tyrosine kinase inhibitor (TKI) of c-KIT. Imatinib has initial response rates of 75–80% [3].

For localized disease, complete resection is the primary treatment and only chance of cure [1, 4]. Although complete resection is possible in 85% of patients, 40% recur within 18–24 months after complete resection [5–7]. Risk of recurrence is associated with increased mitotic rates (>5/50HPFs), tumor size, tumor perforation, and small bowel location [8]. Adjuvant imatinib is recommended for patients with high or intermediate risk.

R.M. Dodson, MD • P. Shen, MD • E.A. Levine, MD
Surgical Oncology, Wake Forest Baptist Health, Winston-Salem, NC, USA

K.I. Votanopoulos, MD, PhD (✉)
Surgical Oncology, Wake Forest Baptist Health, Winston-Salem, NC, USA

Surgical Oncology, Wake Forest University,
Medical Center Blvd, Winston-Salem, North Carolina 27157, USA
e-mail: kvotanop@wakehealth.edu

© Springer International Publishing AG 2017

E. Canbay (ed.), *Unusual Cases in Peritoneal Surface Malignancies*,
DOI 10.1007/978-3-319-51523-6_8

Metastatic disease occurs in 15–47% of patients and most commonly in the liver, peritoneum, and omentum and only rarely in lymph nodes. Extra-abdominal metastasis including the lungs or bone represents advanced disease. In advanced disease that is either unresectable or metastatic, imatinib has significantly improved progression-free survival (PFS) and overall survival (OS). TKIs are the primary treatment of metastatic GISTs. Prior to imatinib, median survival was 10–20 months with a 5-year survival of less than 10%. Imatinib has allowed for median OS of 50–60 months and a 5-year OS of approximately 50% [9].

8.2 Role of Surgery in Metastatic Disease

In selected patients with limited metastatic disease, resection of isolated peritoneal and liver metastasis has shown benefit [10–13]. The National Comprehensive Cancer Network (NCCN) recommends resection in cases of limited disease progression, locally advanced disease, or previously unresectable tumors following a favorable response to treatment. Optimal timing of resection has been disputed in the setting of metastatic disease. There are two strategies that have been recommended. The first, proposed by Haller et al., is to treat with TKI and reserve for surgery until there are signs of resistance [14]. The second strategy employs surgery at least 6 months after the initiation of TKI therapy to maximize the period of responsiveness to TKI and prior to the appearance of resistant disease. This strategy has been employed by DeMatteo et al. from Memorial Sloan Kettering [15]. A multi-institutional study between Duke, Pittsburg, and Johns Hopkins of 39 patients that underwent hepatectomy for metastatic GISTs also supports this approach. In this study, 59% received preoperative TKI, and median duration of imatinib was 18 months. Patients who had >18 months of preoperative TKI had poorer DFS and OS [12]. Receipt of postoperative TKI therapy was associated with significantly improved survival.

Current literature supports resection of responsive disease after 6 months, but prior to 2 years. Waiting at least 6 months has been recommended to allow for maximal response, which typically occurs 6–9 months after initiation of imatinib, and to allow for determination of response to therapy. The response to TKI has significant prognostic value, as patients with disease progression on a TKI will have poor outcomes despite complete resection. At baseline, nearly 14% of patients have primary resistance, and half of patients develop secondary resistance by 2 years. It is therefore also recommended that patients undergo resection by 2 years to avoid resistant clone proliferation. Additionally, patients should resume TKI therapy as early as possible postoperatively, essentially once the patient is able to tolerate oral intake.

8.3 Cytoreductive Surgery (CS)

8.3.1 Pre-imatinib Era

Prior to TKI/imatinib therapy, response rates to standard chemotherapy were extremely low, less than 10%. Complete macroscopic resection (R0/R1) of GISTs was the only chance of obtaining improved survival and cure [16–18]. DeMatteo et al. studied 127 patients from 1983–2002 that underwent complete (R0/R1) resection of primary GISTs [19]. RFS at 1 and 5 years was 83% and 63%, respectively. This Memorial Sloan Kettering Cancer Center (MSKCC) group found the following risk factors for recurrence: ≥5 mitoses/50 high-power fields, tumor size ≥10 cm, and small bowel primary tumor. They also determined that specific KIT mutations had prognostic importance: (1) KIT exon 11 point mutations and insertions had a favorable prognosis, (2) KIT exon 9 mutations and KIT exon 11 deletions had a higher rate of recurrence, and (3) patients without tyrosine kinase mutations had intermediate outcome.

Gold et al. studied 199 patients with metastatic GISTs prior to the use of imatinib [20]. In this retrospective study, 68% of patients with metastatic disease underwent resection with improved overall survival compared to the 42% that underwent conventional chemotherapy only. Median survival for the entire cohort was 19 months, 2-year survival was 41%, and 5-year survival was 25%. In contrast, after imatinib treatment, median survival was extended to 58 months and 2-year survival rates to 72%.

8.3.2 Post-imatinib Era

8.3.2.1 Adjuvant Treatment

Studies of adjuvant imatinib therapy demonstrate decreased risk of recurrence. Duration of adjuvant treatment has been extended from 1 year to 3–5 years for patients with high-risk features. One of the first trials to test adjuvant imatinib was ACOSOG Z9000, which administered imatinib at a dose of 400 mg daily for 12 months to 106 patients [21]. This trial found factors associated with decreased RFS including increasing tumor size, small bowel origin, mitotic rate, age, and KIT exon 9 mutations. ACOSOG Z9001, a phase III double-blinded study, randomized patients with primary localized GISTs to 1 year of postoperative imatinib therapy in 317 patients versus placebo in 328 patients [22]. This study was closed early due to the significantly fewer recurrence events in the imatinib arm. In this study, RFS was improved by imatinib therapy 98% vs 83% in favor of imatinib (HR 0.35, 95% CI,

0.22–0.53). In addition, this study also found that patients with exon 11 deletions had longer RFS on imatinib. The Scandinavian Sarcoma Group (SSGXVIII/AIO) trial compared imatinib therapy at 400 mg daily for 1 year versus 3 years and found that 3 years of therapy was associated with improved RFS and OS in high-risk GISTs, as well as patients with exon 11 mutations [23].

8.3.2.2 Neoadjuvant Treatment

Andtbacka et al. in a retrospective review of 46 patients that were treated with neo-adjuvant imatinib at a dose of 400 mg daily found that imatinib decreased tumor size and was associated with complete resection [10]. This study included 11 patients with primary GISTs and 35 patients with recurrent or metastatic GISTs. All primary GIST patients underwent complete resection, whereas only 11 of the 35 patients with recurrent/metastatic GISTs underwent complete resection. Patients with PR had higher R0/R1 resection rates. The RTOG 0132/ACRIN 6665, a phase II trial of neo-adjuvant imatinib followed by 2 years of adjuvant imatinib, prospectively studied 30 patients with resectable primary GISTs and 22 patients with potentially resectable recurrent or metastatic disease [24]. The authors found 7% PR, 83% SD, 83% PFS, and 93% 2-year OS in patients with primary resectable disease versus 4.5% PR, 91% SD, 77% PFS, and 91% 2-year OS in patients with recurrent/metastatic GISTs. This study was limited to only patients that responded to therapy. The median duration of preoperative imatinib in the recurrent/metastatic group was 2.1 months, which is potentially shorter than that needed to achieve maximal response.

8.3.2.3 Neoadjuvant Therapy for Locally Advanced, Recurrent, and Metastatic Disease

Studies of TKIs in the neoadjuvant setting for metastatic disease are limited and support surgery for limited metastatic disease, disease that demonstrates response to TKI therapy, and disease that can be completely resected [10, 15, 25–28].

1. Bauer et al. reported their European multi-institutional study of preoperative imatinib in 239 patients with metastatic disease [25]. In this study, median duration of preoperative imatinib therapy was 1.1 years, and an R0/R1 was performed in 74% of patients. Patients who had a complete resection had an 8.7-year OS vs 5.3-year OS in patients that had an R2 resection ($P = 0.0001$). PFS in patients with an R2 resection was 1.9 year and had not been reached in R0/R1. The authors conclude that survival benefit can be achieved for metastasectomy if completely resected.
2. Raut et al. reported on a single institutional study of 69 patients with advanced GISTs and their responsiveness to preoperative TKI [28]. R0/R1 was performed in 78% with SD, 25% with limited disease progression (LDP), and 7% in generalized disease progression (GDP). Response to therapy was related to both PFS and OS at 12 months. PFS for SD, LDP, and GDP was 80%, 33%, and 0%,

respectively ($P < 0.001$). OS was 95%, 86%, and 0% for SD, LDP, and GDP, respectively ($P < 0.001$). The authors conclude that cytoreductive surgery has a limited role in patients demonstrating disease progression while on TKI.

3. Gronchi et al. reported a single institution experience from Milan of 37 patients with advanced/metastatic GIST that underwent surgery after imatinib [27]. The authors found that DSS at 12 months was 100% for patients responding to imatinib, whereas DSS was 60% for patients progressing on imatinib. The authors conclude that patients progressing on imatinib do not have major benefit from surgery.

4. DeMatteo et al. reported on 40 patients with metastatic GISTs treated with a median of 15 months of preoperative TKI therapy [15]. Response to therapy was graded as responsive disease, focal resistance (one tumor growing), or multifocal resistance (more than one tumor growing). Overall survival at 2 years for responsive disease was 100%, focal resistance was 61%, and multifocal resistance was 31%. PFS of responsive was 61% at 2 years, focal resistant disease progressed at a median of 12 months, and multifocal resistant disease progressed at a median of 3 months. The authors conclude that patients with metastatic GIST that have responsive disease or focal resistance to TKI can benefit from resection; however, patients with multifocal resistance do not have significant benefit from resection.

5. Zaydfudim et al. reported on a single intuitional experience from the Mayo Clinic of 87 patients with recurrent or metastatic GISTs from 2002 to 2011 [13]. Of these 87 patients, 54 underwent exploration and 36% had R0 resection. TKI was used preoperatively in 32 patients of which 40% had partial response, 31% had stable disease, and 28% had progressive disease. The authors found that OS and PFS were strongly associated with response to TKI and R0 resection (all $P = 0.002$).

6. Bischof et al. reported on a multi-institutional study of 87 patients with locally advanced GISTs and 71 patients with recurrent/metastatic GISTs from 1998 to 2012 [26]. Complete resection was performed in 87% of patients. Preoperative TKI was received by only 56% of patients. Responses were as follows: 5% had a complete response, 49% had a partial response, 28% had stable disease, and 18% had progressive disease. Median OS was 17.1 months for PD and had not yet been reached for patients with SD or PR. The authors conclude (1) that there was underutilization of preoperative TKIs, (2) that high rates of R0 resection could be achieved with preoperative TKI, and (3) that patients who have responsive or stable disease experience improved RFS and OS.

8.4   Cytoreductive Surgery and Hyperthermic Intraperitoneal Chemotherapy (HIPEC)

There are several studies of peritoneal sarcomatosis and the use of cytoreductive surgery combined with HIPEC [29–34]. The role of HIPEC procedures in the management of patients with gastrointestinal stromal tumor (GIST)-induced sarcomatosis is not well defined. Prior to 2002, patients that developed GIST-induced sarcomatosis had limited options as their disease was relatively resistant to standard chemotherapy.

To combat sarcomatosis, a few patients were offered HIPEC. Eilber et al. report on the UCLA Sarcoma Study Group's experience of 46 patients who had cytoreductive surgery with or without post for recurrent GISTs from 1988 to 1998 [33]. Postoperative intraperitoneal therapy with mitoxantrone was used in 33 patients and given in four to six courses at 2–3-week intervals. The median DFS, 1-year recurrence rates, and peritoneal recurrence rates for the cytoreductive alone versus postoperative HIPEC were 8 vs 11 months, 85% vs 52%, and 92% vs 39%, respectively. Liver recurrence rates were similar 85% vs 82% and a key determinate in overall survival.

In a retrospective review by Bryan et al. from 1992 to 2013 of a single institution performance of 1,070 cytoreductive surgeries with HIPEC, only 18 HIPECs were performed for GIST-induced sarcomatosis [35]. These 18 HIPECs were performed on 16 patients. Patients had similar high rates of morbidity (30%) and mortality (5%) following HIPEC as other primaries. Neoadjuvant and/or target therapy was used in 63% of patients, and R0/R1 was achieved in 72% of patients. The midpoint of the study is at the introduction of TKI therapy. Preoperative and/or postoperative TKI therapy was used in 10 out of 16 patients. Although not significant due to low power of the study, the mean survival of patients that received a TKI was 7.89 years versus 1.04 years for patients that did not receive a TKI.

On subgroup analysis of patients that underwent optimal surgical therapy (R0/R1), median survival for patients that did not receive a TKI was 1.09 years versus a median survival that was not yet reached for those that did receive a TKI. Another important finding in this study was that the response to TKI therapy was associated with survival. The median survival for patients that progressed on TKI was 1.35 years after HIPEC versus a median survival that had not yet been reached for patients that did not progress on TKI after HIPEC ($P = 0.007$). In addition, patients that progressed on preoperative TKIs had a higher rate of incomplete resection. The results from this study suggest that the improvement in survival is not related to the HIPEC procedure, but instead to TKI therapy. The authors found that HIPEC could achieve similar long-term survival as that reported from standard cytoreduction without HIPEC.

The subgroup of patients that were referred for HIPEC after progression on TKI did extremely poorly. Therefore, cytoreduction should be performed prior to the development of TKI resistance, as progression on TKI was associated with poor outcomes even when complete cytoreduction could be obtained. In conclusion, the authors support cytoreductive surgery without HIPEC for GIST sarcomatosis when patients have either responsive or stable disease on preoperative imaging to TKI therapy.

References

1. Quek R, George S. Gastrointestinal stromal tumor: a clinical overview. Hematol Oncol Clin N Am. 2009;23:69–78. viii
2. Maki RG, Blay JY, Demetri GD, et al. Key issues in the clinical management of gastrointestinal stromal tumors: an expert discussion. Oncologist. 2015;20:823–30.
3. Scaife CL, Hunt KK, Patel SR, et al. Is there a role for surgery in patients with "unresectable" cKIT+ gastrointestinal stromal tumors treated with imatinib mesylate? Am J Surg. 2003;186:665–9.
4. Gronchi A, Raut CP. The combination of surgery and imatinib in GIST: a reality for localized tumors at high risk, an open issue for metastatic ones. Ann Surg Oncol. 2012;19:1051–5.
5. Chen LL, Trent JC, Wu EF, et al. A missense mutation in KIT kinase domain 1 correlates with imatinib resistance in gastrointestinal stromal tumors. Cancer Res. 2004;64:5913–9.
6. Antonescu CR, Besmer P, Guo T, et al. Acquired resistance to imatinib in gastrointestinal stromal tumor occurs through secondary gene mutation. Clin Cancer Res Off J Am Assoc Cancer Res. 2005;11:4182–90.
7. Heinrich MC, Corless CL, Demetri GD, et al. Kinase mutations and imatinib response in patients with metastatic gastrointestinal stromal tumor. J Clin Oncol. 2003;21:4342–9.
8. McAuliffe JC, Hunt KK, Lazar AJ, et al. A randomized, phase II study of preoperative plus postoperative imatinib in GIST: evidence of rapid radiographic response and temporal induction of tumor cell apoptosis. Ann Surg Oncol. 2009;16:910–9.
9. von Mehren M, Randall RL, Benjamin RS, et al. Soft tissue sarcoma, version 2.2016, NCCN clinical practice guidelines in oncology. J Natl Compr Cancer Netw JNCCN. 2016;14:758–86.
10. Andtbacka RH, Ng CS, Scaife CL, et al. Surgical resection of gastrointestinal stromal tumors after treatment with imatinib. Ann Surg Oncol. 2007;14:14–24.
11. de la Fuente SG, Deneve JL, Parsons CM, Zager JS, Conley AP, Gonzalez RJ. A comparison between patients with gastrointestinal stromal tumours diagnosed with isolated liver metastases and liver metastases plus sarcomatosis. HPB: Off J Int Hepatol Pancreatol Biliary Assoc. 2013;15:655–60.
12. Turley RS, Peng PD, Reddy SK, et al. Hepatic resection for metastatic gastrointestinal stromal tumors in the tyrosine kinase inhibitor era. Cancer. 2012;118:3571–8.
13. Zaydfudim V, Okuno SH, Que FG, Nagorney DM, Donohue JH. Role of operative therapy in treatment of metastatic gastrointestinal stromal tumors. J Surg Res. 2012;177:248–54.
14. Haller F, Detken S, Schulten HJ, et al. Surgical management after neoadjuvant imatinib therapy in gastrointestinal stromal tumours (GISTs) with respect to imatinib resistance caused by secondary KIT mutations. Ann Surg Oncol. 2007;14:526–32.
15. DeMatteo RP, Maki RG, Singer S, Gonen M, Brennan MF, Antonescu CR. Results of tyrosine kinase inhibitor therapy followed by surgical resection for metastatic gastrointestinal stromal tumor. Ann Surg. 2007;245:347–52.
16. Le Cesne A, Judson I, Crowther D, et al. Randomized phase III study comparing conventional-dose doxorubicin plus ifosfamide versus high-dose doxorubicin plus ifosfamide plus recombinant human granulocyte-macrophage colony-stimulating factor in advanced soft tissue sarcomas: a trial of the European Organization for Research and Treatment of Cancer/Soft Tissue and Bone Sarcoma Group. J Clin Oncol. 2000;18:2676–84.
17. Nielsen OS, Judson I, van Hoesel Q, et al. Effect of high-dose ifosfamide in advanced soft tissue sarcomas. A multicentre phase II study of the EORTC Soft Tissue and Bone Sarcoma Group. Eur J Cancer. 2000;36:61–7.

18. Patel SR, Gandhi V, Jenkins J, et al. Phase II clinical investigation of gemcitabine in advanced soft tissue sarcomas and window evaluation of dose rate on gemcitabine triphosphate accumulation. J Clin Oncol. 2001;19:3483–9.
19. Dematteo RP, Gold JS, Saran L, et al. Tumor mitotic rate, size, and location independently predict recurrence after resection of primary gastrointestinal stromal tumor (GIST). Cancer. 2008;112:608–15.
20. Gold JS, van der Zwan SM, Gonen M, et al. Outcome of metastatic GIST in the era before tyrosine kinase inhibitors. Ann Surg Oncol. 2007;14:134–42.
21. DeMatteo RP, Ballman KV, Antonescu CR, et al. Long-term results of adjuvant imatinib mesylate in localized, high-risk, primary gastrointestinal stromal tumor: ACOSOG Z9000 (Alliance) intergroup phase 2 trial. Ann Surg. 2013;258:422–9.
22. Dematteo RP, Ballman KV, Antonescu CR, et al. Adjuvant imatinib mesylate after resection of localised, primary gastrointestinal stromal tumour: a randomised, double-blind, placebo-controlled trial. Lancet. 2009;373:1097–104.
23. Joensuu H, Eriksson M, Sundby Hall K, et al. One vs three years of adjuvant imatinib for operable gastrointestinal stromal tumor: a randomized trial. JAMA. 2012;307:1265–72.
24. Eisenberg BL, Harris J, Blanke CD, et al. Phase II trial of neoadjuvant/adjuvant imatinib mesylate (IM) for advanced primary and metastatic/recurrent operable gastrointestinal stromal tumor (GIST): early results of RTOG 0132/ACRIN 6665. J Surg Oncol. 2009;99:42–7.
25. Bauer S, Rutkowski P, Hohenberger P, et al. Long-term follow-up of patients with GIST undergoing metastasectomy in the era of imatinib – analysis of prognostic factors (EORTC-STBSG collaborative study). Eur J Surg Oncol J Eur Soc Surg Oncol Br Assoc Surg Oncol. 2014;40:412–9.
26. Bischof DA, Kim Y, Blazer 3rd DG, et al. Surgical management of advanced gastrointestinal stromal tumors: an international multi-institutional analysis of 158 patients. J Am Coll Surg. 2014;219:439–49.
27. Gronchi A, Fiore M, Miselli F, et al. Surgery of residual disease following molecular-targeted therapy with imatinib mesylate in advanced/metastatic GIST. Ann Surg. 2007;245:341–6.
28. Raut CP, Posner M, Desai J, et al. Surgical management of advanced gastrointestinal stromal tumors after treatment with targeted systemic therapy using kinase inhibitors. J Clin Oncol. 2006;24:2325–31.
29. Levine EA, Stewart JH, Russell GB, Geisinger KR, Loggie BL, Shen P. Cytoreductive surgery and intraperitoneal hyperthermic chemotherapy for peritoneal surface malignancy: experience with 501 procedures. J Am Coll Surg. 2007;204:943–53. discussion 53–5
30. Randle RW, Swett KR, Shen P, Stewart JH, Levine EA, Votanopoulos KI. Cytoreductive surgery with hyperthermic intraperitoneal chemotherapy in peritoneal sarcomatosis. Am Surg. 2013;79:620–4.
31. Rossi CR, Deraco M, De Simone M, et al. Hyperthermic intraperitoneal intraoperative chemotherapy after cytoreductive surgery for the treatment of abdominal sarcomatosis: clinical outcome and prognostic factors in 60 consecutive patients. Cancer. 2004;100:1943–50.
32. Levine EA, Stewart JH, Shen P, Russell GB, Loggie BL, Votanopoulos KI. Intraperitoneal chemotherapy for peritoneal surface malignancy: experience with 1,000 patients. J Am Coll Surg. 2014;218:573–85.
33. Eilber FC, Rosen G, Forscher C, Nelson SD, Dorey F, Eilber FR. Recurrent gastrointestinal stromal sarcomas. Surg Oncol. 2000;9:71–5.
34. Eilber FC, Rosen G, Forscher C, Nelson SD, Dorey FJ, Eilber FR. Surgical resection and intraperitoneal chemotherapy for recurrent abdominal sarcomas. Ann Surg Oncol. 1999;6:645–50.
35. Bryan ML, Fitzgerald NC, Levine EA, Shen P, Stewart JH, Votanopoulos KI. Cytoreductive surgery with hyperthermic intraperitoneal chemotherapy in sarcomatosis from gastrointestinal stromal tumor. Am Surg. 2014;80:890–5.

Chapter 9
Treatment of Peritoneal Metastases from Breast Cancer by Maximal Cytoreduction and HIPEC

Paolo Sammartino, Maurizio Cardi, Tommaso Cornali, Bianca Maria Sollazzo, Rosa Marcellinaro, Alessio Impagnatiello, and Di Giorgio Angelo

9.1 Introduction

Breast cancer (BC) is the most frequently occurring cancer and the leading cause of cancer death among females worldwide with an estimated 1.7 million cases and more than 500,000 deaths in 2012 [1, 2]. The current 5-year relative survival rates of 97% and 78% for localized and regional disease, respectively, indicate that a significant proportion of BC patients will experience prolonged survival [3]. Although the risk of BC recurrence diminishes over time, late recurrences well into the second decade of surveillance can occur. Metastatic BC represents an important challenge for specialists, and typical metastases sites include, in order of frequency, bones, liver, lungs, and brain. As local and systemic treatments improve, BC metastasis patterns are changing so that metastatic disease now manifests at unusual sites. Peritoneal metastases (PM) have been reported in 0.7% of patients with BC [4], and these patients are typically considered as having a terminal and incurable disease and justifiably treated by palliation with a very poor prognosis. In general, PM are long term confined to the peritoneal cavity without other distant metastasis, and therefore a regional approach seems reasonable in selected patients. No clear guidelines are available regarding the role of cytoreductive surgery (CRS) with or without hyperthermic intraperitoneal chemotherapy (HIPEC) in PM from BC. Over the past two decades, a novel therapeutic approach that combines cytoreductive surgery (CRS) and hyperthermic intraperitoneal chemotherapy (HIPEC) has emerged. This treatment radically changed the outcome of patients with peritoneal surface

P. Sammartino, MD, PhD (✉) • M. Cardi, MD, PhD • T. Cornali, MD • B.M. Sollazzo, MD
R. Marcellinaro, MD • A. Impagnatiello, MD • D.G. Angelo, MD
University of Rome "Sapienza", Department Pietro Valdoni,
Policlinico Umberto I, Viale del Policlinico 155, 00161 Rome, Italy
e-mail: paolo.sammartino@uniroma1.it; maurizio.cardi@uniroma1.it; tommaso.cornali@uniroma1.it; bianca.sollazo@gmail.com; rosamarcellinaro@gmail.com; alessio.impagnatiello@uniroma1.it; angelo.digiorgio@uniroma1.it

© Springer International Publishing AG 2017   111
E. Canbay (ed.), *Unusual Cases in Peritoneal Surface Malignancies*,
DOI 10.1007/978-3-319-51523-6_9

malignancies (PSM) and is now regarded as the standard of care for pseudomyxoma peritonei, peritoneal mesotheliomas, and moderate to small volume PM from colorectal cancers [5–7]. Many studies also reported prolonged survival with this combined approach for the treatment of peritoneal metastases from ovarian and gastric cancers [8, 9]. Expanding literature reports helped to identify not only the primary tumors for which CRS plus HIPEC offer a clear advantage but also those with rare or unusual primary tumors who may benefit from this treatment modality [10–13]. This chapter reports our single-institution experience with CRS plus HIPEC in the treatment of patients with PM from BC.

9.2   Patients and Methods

From the clinical records of 363 patients admitted in our institution from November 2000 to December 2015 with a diagnosis of PM from various primary tumors and treated by maximal CRS and HIPEC with a standardized surgical technique [14], we selected for this retrospective review the patients with a clear histological diagnosis of PM from BC; performance status 0–2 WHO [15]; adequate cardiac, hepatic, renal, and bone marrow function; and resectable disease.

Exclusion criteria were progressive and unresponsive disease, other malignancies, unresectable disease and active infections, or severe associated medical conditions. To rule out the differential diagnosis with other malignancies, PM from BC were assayed with a specific immunohistochemical panel [16].

At laparotomy, the extent of peritoneal spread was recorded using the peritoneal cancer index (PCI) according to Sugarbaker's criteria [17]. Surgical cytoreduction was then undertaken with the aim to leave no macroscopically visible residual disease. The completeness of cytoreduction (CC) score was calculated according to Sugarbaker's criteria [18]. HIPEC was then given with the closed technique [19]: four surgical drains were positioned for inflow/outflow and temperature monitoring and connected to a sterile closed extraperitoneal circuit with up to 6 L of perfusate circulating by means of a peristaltic pump at a flow rate of 500 ml/min. HIPEC was given at temperatures ranging from 42 to 43 °C for 60 min with cisplatin at a dose of 75 mg/m^2. Trendelenburg/anti-Trendelenburg and latero-lateral inclinations were changed every 5 min to guarantee that the whole peritoneal surface would be perfused. As a final step, the abdomen was rinsed with 3–4 L of sterile saline solution at 37 °C.

During the immediate postoperative period, patients were assisted in an ICU unit for at least 24 h. Treatment-related morbidity and mortality were recorded using the Clavien-Dindo classification [20]. Patients were referred to the medical oncologist staff to plan eventual systemic adjuvant chemotherapy. A total body computed tomographic (CT) scan was acquired to evaluate eventual measurable residual disease. Patients with residual disease (CC > 0) were advised to undergo adjuvant systemic treatment, according to tumor biological features (ER, PR, and HER2 expression) and patient clinical conditions. Aromatase inhibitors were used for postmenopausal ER or PR-positive peritoneal disease or both, and patients with HER2-positive tumor expression at histology underwent combination therapy with trastuzumab. Patients with no residual disease (CC0) were advised to undergo adjuvant systemic chemotherapy as a precautional option. Every 6 months, patients underwent assessment of clinical conditions, serum markers, and CT scan findings as well as other diagnostic measures as needed.

9.3 Results

Of the 363 patients who underwent maximal cytoreduction and HIPEC for various primary cancers, we considered for the study seven patients who had a histological diagnosis of peritoneal carcinomatosis from BC. Mean age at cytoreduction and HIPEC was 63.6 years (range 52–77). The clinical characteristics and related treatments are reported in Table 9.1. Immunohistochemical features of the primary BC and peritoneal relapse in the seven patients are reported in Table 9.2.

None of the patients were breast cancer gene (BRCA) mutation carriers, and all patients' tumors tested negative for WT1 and Ca-125 and positive for GCDFP-15. Surgical-related morbidity and mortality are shown in Table 9.3. After receiving HIPEC, one patient experienced a transient grade II cisplatin renal toxicity reversed by medical treatment and one patient a moderate pancreatitis requiring medical treatment. The mean PCI was 19 (range 15–24). Long-term survival is reported in Table 9.4. Of the seven patients, four are presently alive and disease-free at 11, 58, 117, and 135 months.

Table 9.1 Clinical characteristics related to the primary breast cancer

Patient	Age (years)	Histology	Stage	Surgery	Radiotherapy	Adjuvant chemotherapy
Pt 1	58	IDC	T2 N1	Radical mastectomy	No	CMF
Pt 2	54	ILC	T2N3	Quadrantectomy	Yes	Refused
Pt 3	55	ILC	T2 N1 M1 (bone)	Radical mastectomy	No	CMF
Pt 4	77	IDC	T2 N1	Radical mastectomy	No	Refused
Pt 5	53	IDC	T1 N0	Radical mastectomy	No	None
Pt 6	70	ILC	T2N1	Radical mastectomy	Yes	CMF+ H-Th
Pt 7	63	ILC	T2 N0	Radical mastectomy	No	H-Th

IDC infiltrating ductal carcinoma, *ILC* infiltrating lobular carcinoma, *CMF* cyclophosphamide/methotrexate/5-fluorouracil regimen, *H-Th* hormone therapy

Table 9.2 Immunohistochemical panel findings in the seven patients at primary diagnosis and at peritoneal relapse

Patient	BRCA carrier Status	ER PR HER-2 Primary	Relapse	WT1 Primary	Relapse	GCDFP-15 Primary	Relapse	CK7 CK20 Ca-125 Primary	Relapse
Pt 1	Neg	+	+++	Neg	Neg	Neg	+	Pos	Pos
		+	Neg					Neg	Neg
		Neg	Neg					Pos	Neg
Pt 2	Neg	+	+	Neg	Neg	Neg	+	Pos	Pos
		Neg	Neg					Pos	Neg
		+	++					Neg	Neg
Pt 3	Neg	+	++	Neg	Neg	Neg	++	Pos	Pos
		Neg	Neg					Neg	Neg
		Neg	++					Pos	Neg
Pt 4	Neg	Neg	Neg	Neg	Neg	Neg	++	Pos	Pos
		Neg	Neg					Neg	Neg
		Neg	Neg					Neg	Neg
Pt 5	Neg	Neg	++	Neg	Neg	Neg	+++	Pos	Pos
		Neg	+					Neg	Neg
		Neg	Neg					Neg	Neg
Pt 6	Neg	++	++	Neg	Neg	Neg	++	Pos	Pos
		+	+					Neg	Neg
		+	+					Neg	Neg
Pt 7	Neg	+++	++	Neg	Neg	Neg	+++	Pos	Pos
		+++	++					Pos	Pos
		Neg	Neg					Neg	Neg

BRCA breast cancer gene, *ER* estrogen receptors, *PR* progesterone receptors, *HER2* human epidermal growth factor receptor-2, *WT1* Wilms' tumor 1 suppressor gene, *GCDFP-15* gross cystic disease fluid protein, *CK7* cytokeratin-7, *CK20* cytokeratin-20

Table 9.3 Perioperative data

Patient	Postoperative stay (days)	Length of procedure (min)	Blood loss (cc)	ICU stay (h)	Morbidity (grade, type) Clavien-Dindo [20]
Pt 1	16	220	1,300	18	II, wound infection
Pt 2	24	230	2,000	18	–
Pt 3	20	200	1,100	12	IVa, TIA
Pt 4	21	210	1,400	24	II, pleural effusion, wound infection
Pt 5	11	190	600	12	–
Pt 6	14	200	700	15	III-b, anastomotic leakage
Pt 7	13	180	400	17	II, anemia
Mean	17.0	205	1,100	16.6	–

TIA transient ischemic attack, *ICU* intensive care unit

Table 9.4 Cytoreduction and HIPEC in patients with PM from BC – survival and QOL

Patient	Years after breast cancer	Surgery	PCI	CC	Survival (months)	QOL (3 months)
Pt 1	11	PP + total colectomy greater omentectomy	15	0	Alive DF, 135	8.1
Pt 2	30	PP + small bowel resection, greater omentectomy, splenectomy appendectomy	22	1	Alive DF, 117	7.4
Pt 3	21	PP + right colectomy, small bowel resection, greater omentectomy	22	2	Dead, 56 for disease progression	5.3
Pt 4	14	PP +, greater omentectomy, splenectomy, appendectomy	24	1	Dead, 63 for disease progression	6.7
Pt 5	18	Hysteroadnexectomy, greater omentectomy, appendectomy	18	0	Alive DF, 58	7.8
Pt 6	14	Right colectomy, greater omentectomy, splenectomy, bilateral oophorectomy, RUQ peritonectomy	20	1	Alive, 22 with disease progression	7.1
Pt 7	17	PP + left colectomy, hysteroadnexectomy, appendectomy, greater omentectomy	15	0	Alive DF, 11	7.5

PCI peritoneal cancer index, *CC* completeness of cytoreduction, *QOL* quality of life, *PP* pelvic peritonectomy (en bloc removal of uterus, ovaries, rectosigmoid colon, parietal peritonectomy to the transverse umbilical line), *RUQ* right upper quadrant, *DF* disease-free

9.4   Case Presentations

Patient 1 In 1994, this 58-year-old patient underwent a left radical mastectomy for a T2 N1 IDC, followed by six cycles of cyclophosphamide/methotrexate/5-fluorouracil (CMF). In September 2004, an ovarian mass and peritoneal carcinomatosis developed with ascites, nodules on the Douglas pouch, bilateral ovarian masses, malignant disease infiltrating the rectum and left colon, and diffuse small nodules on the transverse and right colon (PCI 15). Her ECOG performance status was 1. The patient underwent pelvic peritonectomy, total colectomy with ileorectal anastomoses, greater omentectomy, and HIPEC (CC0). An aromatase inhibitor was prescribed for 5 years. The patient is alive and has been disease-free for more than 11 years.

Patient 2 This 54-year-old woman underwent a left radical mastectomy for T2 N1 ILC in 1997 and refused adjuvant chemotherapy. In March 2006, she was referred to our Institution to investigate ascites. The diagnostic workup disclosed a bilateral ovarian mass and peritoneal carcinomatosis. Laparotomy showed peritoneal disease involving the pouch, omentum, right and sigmoid colon, small bowel, and spleen (PCI 22). Her ECOG performance status was 1. The patient underwent pelvic peritonectomy, right colectomy omentectomy, splenectomy, multiple ablation procedures for small scattered small bowel and mesenteric implants, and HIPEC (CC1). Immunohistochemistry disclosed an HER2-positive tumor (++), and the patient underwent a 2-year treatment course with Herceptin (trastuzumab) and hormone therapy combined. In January 2014, she underwent the ablation of a spinal meningioma. She is currently alive with no evidence of disease at nearly 10 years follow-up.

Patient 3 In 1986, this 52-year-old woman underwent a radical mastectomy for T2 N1 M1 (bone) ILC followed by adjuvant chemotherapy with CMF. In May 2007, she was admitted in emergency for intestinal obstruction. At operation, she was found to have peritoneal carcinomatosis involving the omentum, bilateral ovarian masses, implants of the small bowel and ascending colon, and ascites (PCI 22). Her ECOG performance status was 2. The patient underwent pelvic peritonectomy, right colectomy, small bowel resection, and omentectomy. Scattered small peritoneal implants in the pouch, lateral colic gutters, and small bowel mesentery were ablated by argon beam coagulation. Visible residual disease <2.5 cm was left in the pelvis attached to the presacral fascia (CC2). HIPEC was given to prevent ascites developing. HER2 testing was positive (++), and the patient underwent a 2-year treatment course with Herceptin combined with hormone therapy. In 2009, the patient experienced progressive disease and died in December 2011.

Patient 4 This 77-year-old woman underwent a left upper quadrantectomy and lymph node dissection for a T2 N1 IDC in 1994. After operation, she refused adjuvant chemo and radiotherapy. In 2008, an ovarian mass developed with peritoneal carcinomatosis and bilateral uveitis with hypopyon, considered as an immune response to the concurrent tumor and successfully treated with corticosteroid therapy. Laparotomy disclosed diffuse peritoneal disease including the omentum, bilateral ovarian masses, Douglas pouch, bilateral latero-colic gutters, small bowel mesentery, and splenic hilum, with no ascites (PCI 24). Her ECOG performance status was 1. The patient underwent pelvic peritonectomy, appendectomy, omentectomy, splenectomy, and HIPEC (CC1). Considering her age and biological tumor features, no adjuvant treatment was proposed. At 45 months, the patient showed a supraclavicular LN recurrence. Histology at excisional biopsy confirmed the BC origin. In February 2014, the patient developed peritoneal recurrence and underwent palliative treatment. She died for disease in May 2014.

Patient 5 This 71-year-old woman underwent a left radical mastectomy for a T1 N0, IDC in 1993. About 18 years later, in February 2011, she was referred to our Institution to investigate a bilateral ovarian mass and peritoneal carcinomatosis. At operation, no ascites was found, and metastatic disease involved ovaries, the omentum, pouch, pelvic peritoneum, and small bowel mesentery (PCI 18). Her ECOG performance status was 0. The patient underwent total hysterectomy, bilateral oophorectomy, appendectomy, omentectomy, multiple ablation procedures for small scattered small bowel, and mesenteric implants followed by HIPEC, leaving no visible residual disease (CC0). She received an aromatase inhibitor and is alive and disease-free at 5 years.

Patient 6 In 1999, this 70-year-old patient underwent a left radical mastectomy for T2 N1 ILC followed by adjuvant chemotherapy (CMF) + hormone therapy + radiotherapy for 5 years. In 2013, a retro-orbital mass (metastasis of breast cancer) was treated with CyberKnife, and bone metastases at cervical spine (C7) were palliated by radiotherapy. In February 2014, she was admitted in our department in emergency for intestinal obstruction. At operation, we found peritoneal metastases involving the ascending colon, greater omentum, bilateral ovarian masses, the spleen, and small bowel implants. PCI score was 20. Her ECOG performance status was 2. The patient underwent bilateral oophorectomy, omentectomy, right colectomy, splenectomy, and multiple ablation procedures for small implants in the small bowel and mesentery. Visible residual disease was <2.5 mm (CC1). She received adjuvant chemotherapy for six more cycles, and she is actually alive with disease.

Patient 7 This 63-year-old woman underwent a right radical mastectomy for a T2 N0 ILC in 1998. She had been treated with tamoxifen for 5 years subsequent to her mastectomy. About 17 years later, in January 2015, she was admitted in our department with a CT scan showing ascites and omental and peritoneal implants in the left paracolic gutter at the rectosigmoid junction. Her ECOG performance status was 1. After a laparoscopic procedure and biopsies confirming the mammary origin, the patient underwent a Hartmann procedure, a hysterectomy and bilateral oophorectomy, omentectomy, appendectomy, and pelvic peritonectomy. PCI score was 15. At the end of the procedure, she was left with no macroscopic residual disease (CC0). Immunohistochemistry showed an ER and PR-positive tumor, and she was subsequently continued on hormone therapy. She is presently alive and disease-free at 1 year.

9.5 Discussion

Peritoneal metastases from BC are relatively uncommon but are a great challenge for both medical and surgical oncologists. They include a spectrum of disease ranging from microscopic disease found incidentally at the time of surgery for other indications to widespread symptomatic intraperitoneal metastases. It is reported that about 19% of women dying from nongenital and nonhematologic malignancies have ovarian metastases at autopsy [21], breast cancer representing the single most common nongenital solid tumor metastasizing to the ovary [22], while gastrointestinal metastases are reported to occur in 4–18% of patients with known disseminated BC [23]. Moreover, Curtin et al. found that in 121 women with BC subsequently developing an adnexal mass, 50% were benign and 50% were malignant [24]. Of the malignant cases, 27% were due to metastatic BC, and the remaining 73% were primary ovarian or tubal cancers. This suggests that approximately one in four women with BC that develop a malignant adnexal mass will have intraperitoneal spread. BC is one of the most slowly growing solid tumors, and metastases may appear many years, even decades, after the initial diagnosis [23, 25]. In our patients, a median of 18 years (range 11–30) elapsed between primary BC and PM. This lengthy time lapse accords with other published series describing an interval reaching up to 30 years [25–27]. Considering the increasing number of women with BC and the more protracted disease course, it is likely that the number of women requiring intervention for intraperitoneal breast cancer will increase.

A sensitive factor in assessing women with intraperitoneal BC is confirming tumor pathology, given the increased risk of ovarian cancer in women with BC. In our study, the histopathological reports allowed us to compare the features for the primary BC and the metastatic cancer. As reported by other authors [28], the panel of immunohistochemical stains showing combined negative WT1 and Ca 125 tumor expression associated with positive GCDFP-15 expression in the peritoneal disease invariably strengthened the diagnosis. WT1 is a tumor-suppressor gene that is positive in over 90% of primary ovarian tumors [29] and never found in primary or metastatic BC. Ca 125 is a glycoprotein expressed in up to 90% of ovarian malignancies and from 10% to 30% of primary BC [30]. GCDFP-15 is a relatively specific and sensitive marker for BC (expressed in about 50% of the cases) [31], and never in ovarian malignancies [28].

During the last decades, the progress in loco-regional treatments allowed a significant improvement in breast metastases control. The development of targeted biological drugs against some specific BC subtypes, the possibility of using bone cement to treat destructive bone metastases, the use of interventional radiological techniques in liver metastases, minimally invasive surgery against lung lesions, and the use of gamma knife in brain metastases are just some examples. Our study provides therefore previously unavailable information about the control of intraperitoneal BC spread with cytoreductive surgery and HIPEC. Using this combined approach, of the seven patients treated, five achieved long-term survival, two of them surviving even for 10 years. Moreover, four are alive and disease-free after cytoreduction with maximal residual disease <2.5 mm (CC 1) and after adjuvant chemotherapy.

Unlike gynecologic malignancies, to date no clear guidelines are available for the surgical treatment of intraperitoneal metastatic BC, and surgeons are often faced with the dilemma of whether to proceed with an aggressive debulking of all visible disease when an intraoperative diagnosis of metastatic BC is suspected or confirmed by frozen sections. In a study investigating the role of aggressive surgery for managing metastatic malignancies to the ovaries, Ayhan et al. noted a better mean survival rate (39 vs. 23 months; P = ns) advancing from biopsy alone to aggressive debulking [32]. In 1997, Abu-Rustum et al. reported on 40 patients with metachronous intraperitoneal BC. The median survival for all patients was 24.1 months, and examining the influence of residual disease, although not statistically significant, they noted a trend toward a better survival in patients left with no gross residual disease: 41.6% compared with 16.1% and 18.6% in patients left with gross residual disease (<2 and >2 cm, respectively) [25]. In 2003, Eitan et al. reexamined the role of surgical resection on 59 women with intraperitoneal BC as an update to the report of Abu-Rustum et al. Once again, they found that the amount of disease left in the abdomen was a factor influencing survival, reaching clinical but not statistical significance, with patients who had no residual disease at the end of surgery enjoying a survival benefit (54 vs. 21 months), as well as with those patients who were optimally debulked to less than 2 cm (36 vs. 20 months). Moreover, they found that the presence of metastases outside the abdomen was not a factor that should influence the decision on whether to perform debulking surgery or not [33]. In 2010, Bigorie et al. reported their experience with 29 patients affected by peritoneal spread from BC. At a median follow-up of 2 years, the median global survival was 3 years (range 0.5–9 years), and statistical significance was reached in a comparison between patients who underwent nonoptimal cytoreduction (median survival 2 years) and patients in which was reached an optimal cytoreduction (median survival not reached; $p = 0.015$) [34].

After maximal cytoreduction and HIPEC, morbidity and mortality rates in our patients were in line with those reported for similar procedures [35]. Three patients experienced grade II complications reversed by medical treatment, one patient had a grade III complication (anastomotic leakage) requiring surgical intervention, and one patient had a grade IVa complication (TIA) requiring readmittance in ICU.

Cytoreduction and HIPEC is already regarded as the standard of care in patients with peritoneal metastases from pseudomyxoma peritonei [5], peritoneal mesotheliomas [6], and moderate to small volume colorectal PM [7], and it is also providing promising results from various other primary cancers such as ovary [8] and stomach [9]. Cisplatin is one of the most used chemotherapy agent for HIPEC [36]. In the management of untreated and pretreated metastatic BC, patients with intravenous platinum compounds (cisplatin and carboplatin) have shown activity both as single agents and in combination regimens [37, 38]. Considering its well-known systemic activity and its proved safety in HIPEC technique also reported in our previous experience [19], cisplatin has been considered the drug of choice for our limited series of PM from BC treated with cytoreduction and HIPEC. In conclusion, the long disease-free and overall survival observed in our small series suggests that in highly selected patients in whom surgery can achieve adequate cytoreduction, this combined procedure is a promising approach for patients with peritoneal metastases from BC. From the results of this study, it is not possible to state whether survival in our patients depended on cytoreduction, HIPEC, or both [39] or do our findings indicate the need for adjuvant systemic chemotherapy. These issues warrant further investigations in larger studies.

Conflict of Interest No conflict of interest to disclose.

References

1. Torre LA, Bray F, Siegel RL, Ferlay J, Lortet-Tieulent J, Jemal A. Global cancer statistics, 2012. CA Cancer J Clin. 2015;65(2):87–108.
2. Tao Z, Shi A, Lu C, Song T, Zhang Z, Zhao J. Breast cancer: epidemiology and etiology. Cell Biochem Biophys. 2015;72(2):333–8.
3. American Cancer Society. Cancer facts and figures: American Cancer Society, Inc. 2003. Available at http://www.cancer.org/downloads/stt/caff2003pwsecured.pdf.
4. Bertozzi S, Londero AP, Cedolini C, Uzzau A, Seriau L, Bernardi S, et al. Prevalence, risk factors, and prognosis of peritoneal metastasis from breast cancer. Springerplus. 2015;4:688.
5. Chua TC, Moran BJ, Sugarbaker PH, Levine EA, Glehen O, Gilly FN, et al. Early- and long-term outcome data of patients with pseudomyxoma peritonei from appendiceal origin treated by a strategy of cytoreductive surgery and hyperthermic intraperitoneal chemotherapy. J Clin Oncol. 2012;30(20):2449–56.
6. Yan TD, Deraco M, Baratti D, Kusamura S, Elias D, Glehen O, et al. Cytoreductive surgery and hyperthermic intraperitoneal chemotherapy for malignant peritoneal mesothelioma: multi-institutional experience. J Clin Oncol. 2009;27(36):6237–42.
7. Elias D, Gilly F, Boutitie F, Quenet F, Bereder JM, Mansvelt B, et al. Peritoneal colorectal carcinomatosis treated with surgery and perioperative intraperitoneal chemotherapy: retrospective analysis of 523 patients from a multicentric French study. J Clin Oncol. 2010;28(1):63–8.
8. Bakrin N, Bereder JM, Decullier E, Classe JM, Msika S, Lorimier G, et al. Peritoneal carcinomatosis treated with cytoreductive surgery and hyperthermic intraperitoneal chemotherapy (HIPEC) for advanced ovarian carcinoma: a French multicentre retrospective cohort study of 566 patients. Eur J Surg Oncol. 2013;39(12):1435–43.
9. Yang XJ, Huang CQ, Suo T, Mei LJ, Yang GL, Cheng FL, et al. Cytoreductive surgery and hyperthermic intraperitoneal chemotherapy improves survival of patients with peritoneal carcinomatosis from gastric cancer: final results of a phase III randomized clinical trial. Ann Surg Oncol. 2011;18(6):1575–81.
10. Elias D, David A, Sourrouille I, Honoré C, Goéré D, Dumont F, et al. Neuroendocrine carcinomas: optimal surgery of peritoneal metastases (and associated intra-abdominal metastases). Surgery. 2014;155(1):5–12.
11. Baratti D, Pennacchioli E, Kusamura S, Fiore M, Balestra MR, Colombo C, et al. Peritoneal sarcomatosis: is there a subset of patients who may benefit from cytoreductive surgery and hyperthermic intraperitoneal chemotherapy? Ann Surg Oncol. 2010;17(12):3220–8.
12. Kallianpur AA, Shukla NK, Deo SV, Yadav P, Mudaly D, Yadav R, et al. Updates on the multimodality management of desmoplastic small round cell tumor. J Surg Oncol. 2012;105(6):617–21.
13. Cardi M, Sammartino P, Mingarelli V, Sibio S, Accarpio F, Biacchi D, et al. Cytoreduction and HIPEC in the treatment of "unconventional" secondary peritoneal carcinomatosis. World J Surg Oncol. 2015;13:305.
14. Sugarbaker PH. Peritonectomy procedures. Ann Surg. 1995;221(1):29–42.
15. Oken MM, Creech RH, Tormey DC, Horton J, Davis TE, McFadden ET, et al. Toxicity and response criteria of the Eastern Cooperative Oncology Group. Am J Clin Oncol. 1982;5(6):649–55.
16. Cardi M, Sammartino P, Framarino ML, Biacchi D, Cortesi E, Sibio S, et al. Treatment of peritoneal carcinomatosis from breast cancer by maximal cytoreduction and HIPEC: a preliminary report on 5 cases. Breast. 2013;22(5):845–9.
17. Jacquet P, Sugarbaker PH. Clinical research methodologies in diagnosis and staging of patients with peritoneal carcinomatosis. Cancer Treat Res. 1996;82:359–74.
18. Sugar Baker PH. In: Sugarbaker PH, editor. Peritoneal carcinomatosis. Principles of management. Boston: Kluwer Academic; 1996.

19. Di Giorgio A, Naticchioni E, Biacchi D, Sibio S, Accarpio F, Rocco M, et al. Cytoreductive surgery (peritonectomy procedures) combined with hyperthermic intraperitoneal chemotherapy (HIPEC) in the treatment of diffuse peritoneal carcinomatosis from ovarian cancer. Cancer. 2008;113(2):315–25.
20. Dindo D, Demartines N, Clavien PA. Classification of surgical complications: a new proposal with evaluation in a cohort of 6336 patients and results of a survey. Ann Surg. 2004;240(2):205–13.
21. Fujiwara K, Ohishi Y, Koike H, Sawada S, Moriya T, Kohno I. Clinical implications of metastases to the ovary. Gynecol Oncol. 1995;59(1):124–8.
22. Webb MJ, Decker DG, Mussey E. Cancer metastatic to the ovary: factors influencing survival. Obstet Gynecol. 1975;45(4):391–6.
23. Sheen-Chen SM, Liu YW, Sun CK, Lin SE, Eng HL, Huang WT, et al. Abdominal carcinomatosis attributed to metastatic breast carcinoma. Dig Dis Sci. 2008;53(11):3043–5.
24. Curtin JP, Barakat RR, Hoskins WJ. Ovarian disease in women with breast cancer. Obstet Gynecol. 1994;84(3):449–52.
25. Abu-Rustum NR, Aghajanian CA, Venkatraman ES, Feroz F, Barakat RR. Metastatic breast carcinoma to the abdomen and pelvis. Gynecol Oncol. 1997;66(1):41–4.
26. Nazareno J, Taves D, Preiksaitis HG. Metastatic breast cancer to the gastrointestinal tract: a case series and review of the literature. World J Gastroenterol. 2006;12(38):6219–24.
27. McLemore EC, Pockaj BA, Reynolds C, Gray RJ, Hernandez JL, Grant CS, et al. Breast cancer: presentation and intervention in women with gastrointestinal metastasis and carcinomatosis. Ann Surg Oncol. 2005;12(11):886–94.
28. Tornos C, Soslow R, Chen S, Akram M, Hummer AJ, Abu-Rustum N, et al. Expression of WT1, CA 125, and GCDFP-15 as useful markers in the differential diagnosis of primary ovarian carcinomas versus metastatic breast cancer to the ovary. Am J Surg Pathol. 2005;29(11):1482–9.
29. Silberstein GB, Van Horn K, Strickland P, Roberts Jr CT, Daniel CW. Altered expression of the WT1 wilms tumor suppressor gene in human breast cancer. Proc Natl Acad Sci U S A. 1997;94(15):8132–7.
30. Chhieng DC, Rodriguez-Burford C, Talley LI, Sviglin H, Stockard CR, Kleinberg MJ, et al. Expression of CEA, Tag-72, and Lewis-Y antigen in primary and metastatic lesions of ovarian carcinoma. Hum Pathol. 2003;34(10):1016–21.
31. Wick MR, Lillemoe TJ, Copland GT, Swanson PE, Manivel JC, Kiang DT. Gross cystic disease fluid protein-15 as a marker for breast cancer: immunohistochemical analysis of 690 human neoplasms and comparison with alpha-lactalbumin. Hum Pathol. 1989;20(3):281–7.
32. Ayhan A, Tuncer ZS, Bükülmez O. Malignant tumors metastatic to the ovaries. J Surg Oncol. 1995;60(4):268–76.
33. Eitan R, Gemignani ML, Venkatraman ES, Barakat RR, Abu-Rustum NR. Breast cancer metastatic to abdomen and pelvis: role of surgical resection. Gynecol Oncol. 2003;90(2):397–401.
34. Bigorie V, Morice P, Duvillard P, Antoine M, Cortez A, Flejou JF, et al. Ovarian metastases from breast cancer: report of 29 cases. Cancer. 2010;116(4):799–804.
35. Baratti D, Kusamura S, Mingrone E, Balestra MR, Laterza B, Deraco M. Identification of a subgroup of patients at highest risk for complications after surgical cytoreduction and hyperthermic intraperitoneal chemotherapy. Ann Surg. 2012;256(2):334–41.
36. Chan DL, Morris DL, Rao A, Chua TC. Intraperitoneal chemotherapy in ovarian cancer: a review of tolerance and efficacy. Cancer Manag Res. 2012;4:413–22.
37. Decatris MP, Sundar S, O'Byrne KJ. Platinum-based chemotherapy in metastatic breast cancer: current status. Cancer Treat Rev. 2004;30(1):53–81.
38. Shamseddine AI, Farhat FS. Platinum-based compounds for the treatment of metastatic breast cancer. Chemotherapy. 2011;57(6):468–87.
39. Elias D. Is intraperitoneal chemotherapy after cytoreductive surgery efficient? Knowing whether it is or not appears secondary! Ann Surg Oncol. 2012;19(1):5–6.

Chapter 10
Benign Types of Peritoneal Mesothelioma

Emel Canbay and Yutaka Yonemura

10.1   Introduction

Management of diffuse malignant peritoneal mesothelioma (DMPM) has been explained in our previous book, *Peritoneal Surface Malignancies: A curative Approach* [1]. In this book, we captured on management of rare peritoneal surface malignancies in unusual cases.

Benign multicystic peritoneal mesothelioma (BMPM), well-differentiated papillary peritoneal mesothelioma (WDPPM), and benign adenomatoid mesothelioma (BAM) are the common types of benign peritoneal mesothelioma that are extremely rare tumours originate from peritoneal mesothelial cells. There is no consensus statement for management of these diseases. Many consider cytoreductive surgery (CRS) as a standard of care for benign types of peritoneal mesothelioma. However, a high rate of local recurrence [2] and malignant potential [3, 4] make these tumours potentially target to treat with CRS and hyperthermic intraoperative intraperitoneal chemotherapy (HIPEC).

This report will be structured as a basic knowledge for benign types of peritoneal mesothelioma. Then, integration of CRS and HIPEC into the management of benign types of peritoneal mesothelioma will be reviewed.

E. Canbay, MD, PhD (✉)
NPO HIPEC ISTANBUL, Centre for Peritoneal Surface Oncology,
Guzelbahce Sokak No:15, Istanbul, Turkey
e-mail: drecanbay@gmail.com

Y. Yonemura, MD, PhD
NPO Centre for Peritoneal Surface Oncology, Osaka, Japan

© Springer International Publishing AG 2017   123
E. Canbay (ed.), *Unusual Cases in Peritoneal Surface Malignancies*,
DOI 10.1007/978-3-319-51523-6_10

10.1.1   Benign Multicystic Peritoneal Mesothelioma

Benign multicystic peritoneal mesothelioma (BMPM; peritoneal inclusion cyst, multilocular inclusion cyst, and benign multicystic mesothelioma) is a very rare multilocular cystic tumour which arises from the peritoneal mesothelium [5, 6]. BMPM was first described by Plaut in 1928, and then its mesothelial nature was identified by Mennemeyer and Smith in 1979 [7]. BMPM represents only 3–5% of peritoneal mesotheliomas (PM), whose incidence is 1 per 1,000,000 [8]. BMPM is an exceedingly rare disease that makes its origin, pathogenesis, diagnosis, and management challenging.

Benign multicystic peritoneal mesothelioma (BMPM) usually originates from the pelvic visceral peritoneal mesothelial cells but may develop from intraperitoneal and retroperitoneal areas [9]. This disease usually affects women of reproductive age and shows indolent clinical behaviour [5]. Natural history of development of BMPM is unclear, but previous abdominal surgery or pelvic inflammatory disease has been described [5]. There is no history of asbestos exposure for development of BMPM.

The clinical and imaging features vary among these subtypes of benign type of peritoneal mesothelioma (Table 10.1) [9]. The pathogenesis of BMPM is unknown; malignant transformation or reactive nature has been considered [3, 5, 6]. Malignant transformation is not certain due to the lack of long-term follow-up data as previously reported [3].

Table 10.1   Clinical features of benign type of peritoneal mesotheliomas [9]

Type of benign mesothelioma			
Characteristics	Benign multicystic mesothelioma	Well-differentiated papillary mesothelioma	Benign adenomatoid type of mesothelioma
Predilection	Young to middle-aged women	Reproductive age women	Reproductive age women and men
Predisposing factor	Previous surgery or pelvic inflammatory disease	Not known	Not known
Clinical course	Hormone sensitive	Indolent course, rare malignant change	Indolent course, rare malignant change
Computerized tomography imaging	Multilocular cystic mass, multiple unilocular thin walled cysts, or unilocular cystic mass	Peritoneal thickening, multiple peritoneal nodules, omental infiltration, and ascites	Non-specific
Differential diagnosis	Cystic lymphangioma Endometriosis Cystic epithelial neoplasms of the ovaries Pseudomyxoma peritonei	Peritoneal metastases Serous papillary carcinoma of peritoneum Tuberculous peritonitis	Solid type of metastatic intraperitoneal and retroperitoneal tumours Testicular tumours

10.2 Diagnosis

Most patients are diagnosed incidentally, and clinical findings are also non-specific such as nausea, vomiting, and abdominal pain. However, retroperitoneal mass [10] or acute abdomen due to incisional incarcerated hernia [11] could also be developed in some cases. The palpable fixed mass always presents with tenderness on physical examination. We have reported a case with an incisional hernia, an abdominal discomfort, and a mass surrounded to the umbilicus due to BMPM [12].

Laboratory findings are non-specific for diagnosis of BMPM. An association between BMPM and increased serum CA 19–9 concentration has been described, and a minimally invasive laparoscopic approach enabled both diagnosis and surgical treatment of the disease [13].

Imaging features vary according to the appearance of this tumour. BMPM usually consists multiple cysts but it could be unilocular. Multiseptated cysts can be demonstrated by ultrasonography. However, computerized tomography (CT) is necessary to provide information about the extent and anatomic localization of the disease (Fig. 10.1). In some cases, the omentum can be invaded with multicystic mesothelioma. In our previous report, an intraperitoneal hypodense cystic mass surrounded the umbilicus and extended between the great curvature of the stomach, spleen, and tail of the pancreas extending caudally to the upper margin of the pelvis and resulted with hernia from midline incision scar with CT (Fig. 10.2) [12].

BMPM can also be determined with magnetic resonance imaging (MRI) that shows hypointense well-defined lesions on T1-weighted images and isointense clear watery fluid as intermediate signal intensity on T2-weighted images [14].

Radiological differential diagnosis is made with cystic lymphangioma, cystic epithelial neoplasms of the ovaries [9]. Pseudomyxoma peritonei may rarely resemble BMPM.

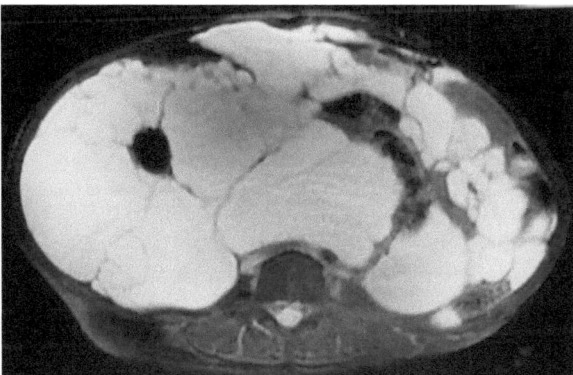

Fig. 10.1 T2-weighted coronal MRI image shows multiloculated cysts which occupied nearly the entire abdominal cavity and omental metastasis of BMPM. Cysts are noncommunicating in abdominal viscera but scalloping to small bowel and its mesentery

Fig. 10.2 Computed tomography images of the BMPM: the *arrows* indicate the incisional hernia (*A*), multicystic mass surrounded to umbilicus (*B*), and intraabdominal extension (*C*)

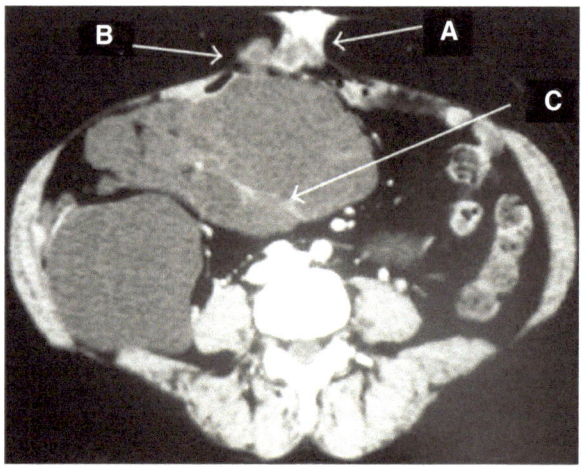

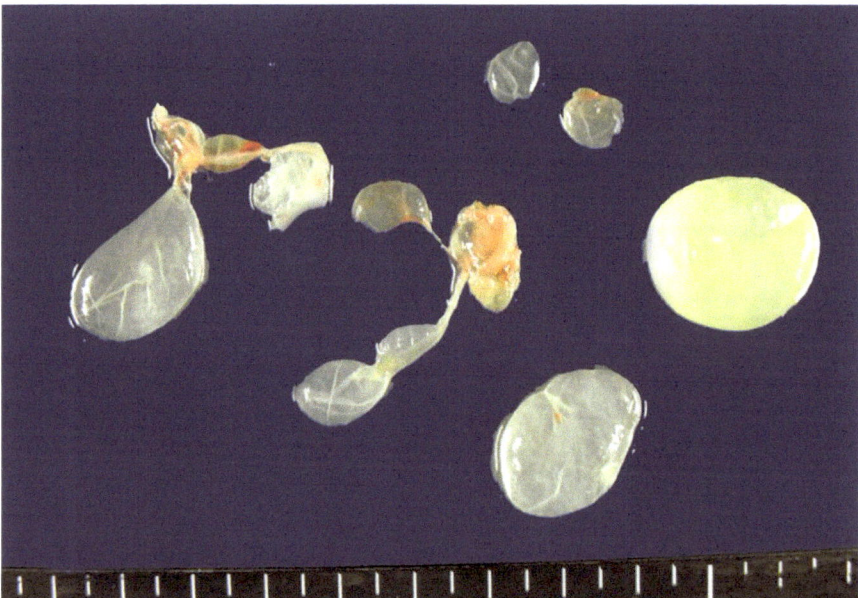

Fig. 10.3 Peritoneal floating cysts (*) and cysts connect with thin stalk to the peritoneal surface

Because BMPM is extremely rare disease, preoperative diagnosis is also challenging. Laparoscopy remains the best diagnostic method that enables to establish the definitive diagnosis with obtaining biopsy. Therefore, we recommend diagnostic laparoscopy and laparoscopic biopsy both from cystic fluid and from tissue specimens.

Multiple floating cysts (Fig. 10.3), widespread multicystic nodular thickening of the visceral peritoneum (Figs. 10.4, 10.5, and 10.6), can be determined during laparotomy or laparoscopic exploration.

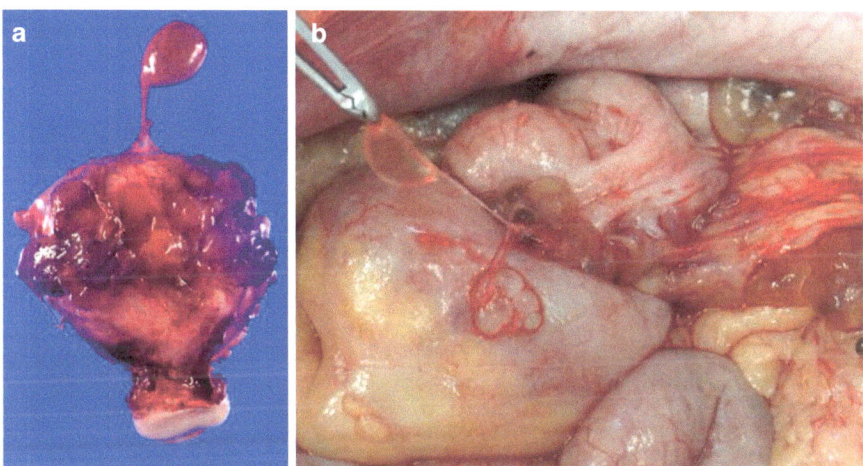

Fig. 10.4 (**a**) Resected BMPM showing multiple fluid-filled cysts on the uterus. Cysts connected with fine stalks from uterine surface. (**b**) Cysts are connected with serosal surface of the visceral organs and omentum

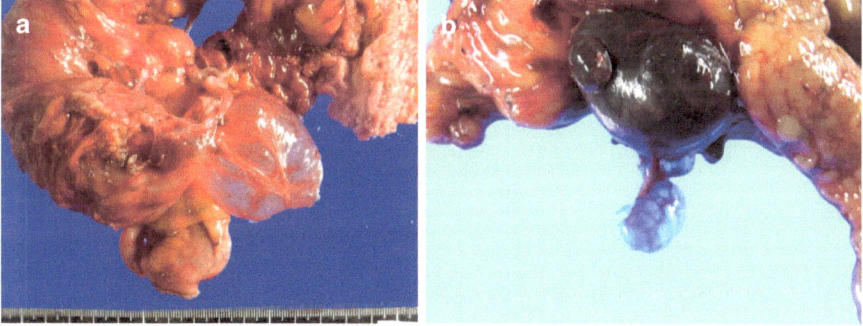

Fig. 10.5 Resected multicystic mesothelioma showing fluid-filled cysts on the caecum (**a**). Cyst was also found on greater omentum with haemorrhagic fluid (**b**)

10.3   Pathology

BMPM is a localized tumour arising from mesothelial cells. Pathological evaluation of BMPM shows that the tumour is composed of a multiple mesothelial-lined cystic structure containing thin watery secretions and lined by a single layer of mesothelial-like cells. Immunohistochemical analysis revealed positive expression of mesothelial cells (Fig. 10.7), calretinin (Fig. 10.8).

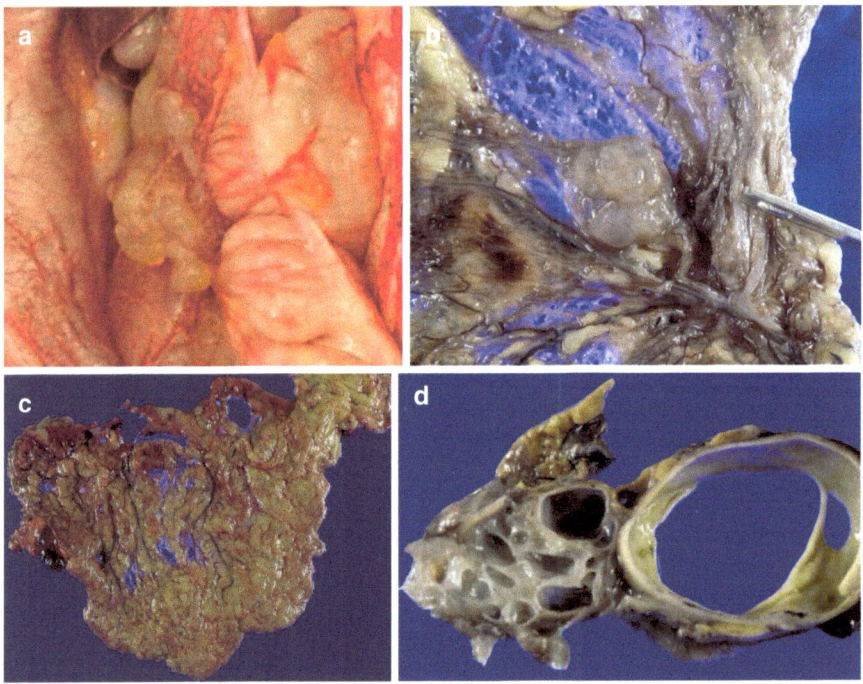

Fig. 10.6 (**a**) Cysts on greater omentum above the hepatic flexure of the colon and (**b, c**) BMPM in greater omentum. (**d**) The cysts are connected with colonic serosa

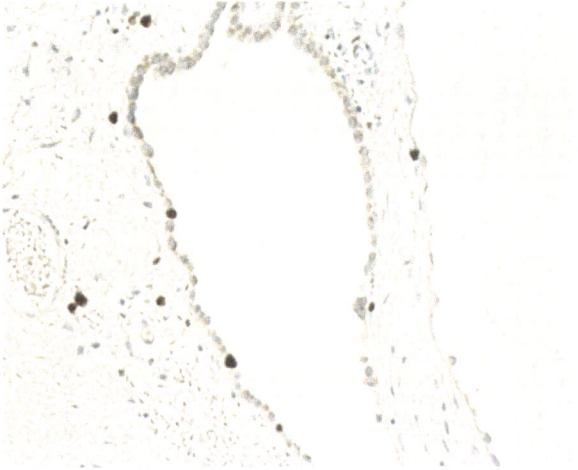

Fig. 10.7 Anti-Ki-67 antibody immunoreaction of cuboidal mesothelial cells lined on the inner surface of cysts (×100)

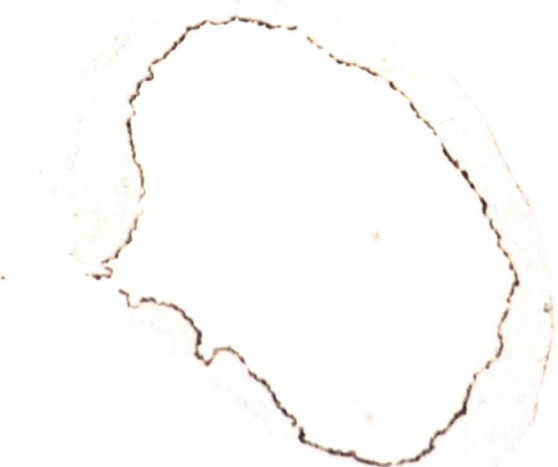

Fig. 10.8 Positive immunoreaction to anti-mesothelin antibody was detected on mesothelial-like cells in inner surface of peritoneal floating cyst (×100)

10.4   Management of BMPM

Surgery remains the mainstay of treatment with complete removal of the cystic lesions to avoid local recurrence even though there are no evidence-based treatment strategies for BMPM. Even the complete removal of the disease, high recurrence rates [15, 16] and malignant transformation [3, 4] have been reported. There is only two series of BMPM treated with aggressive surgery followed by heated intraperitoneal chemotherapy (HIPEC) [17, 18].

In first report, five cases of BMPM, four females and one male, were reviewed by Sethna et al [17]. All patients were symptomatic, and in one patient prolonged conservative treatment for over 10 years resulted with transformation to the invasiveness with lymph node metastasis. Disease control of both ascites and pain in the abdomino-pelvic region was achieved in all patients treated with cytoreductive surgery with HIPEC. They concluded that BMPM should no longer be referred to as "benign" cystic mesothelioma and an aggressive treatment approach with complete disease eradication is the correct goal of treatment.

In second report, four patient of BMPM were reviewed by Baratti et al. [18]. All patients were symptomatic and recurrent cases. Disease control was achieved in three patients treated with cytoreductive surgery with HIPEC. One patient had a recurrence of BMPM and underwent to second-time cytoreductive surgery and HIPEC. They concluded that complete cytoreduction and HIPEC were more effective in preventing recurrence and transformation to malignancy of BMPM.

In our experience (unpublished data), we have eight recurrent patients with BMPM. Of those, one of them has recurrent case of BMPM with incisional hernia [12]. We have performed complete cytoreductive surgery and HIPEC to these patients. So far, none of them had a recurrence or malignant transformation.

These results suggest that cytoreductive surgery to remove all visible tumour and heated intraoperative intraperitoneal chemotherapy to control microscopic residual disease will help patients with BMPM to remain disease-free and to obtain long overall survival with a single surgical intervention.

Disease eradication may prevent the transition to an aggressive and fatal disease process.

Hormonal therapy, sclerotherapy, and thermotherapy as other treatment options have not been proven to provide therapeutic effects for management of BMPM.

The prognosis is excellent. In one of the largest series reported by Weiss and Tavassoli [5], only two cases of death were reported [5].

The observation of malignant transformation mandates systematic clinical follow-up of these patients. Further follow-up is compounded by the fact that there are no reliable clinical or imaging features or tumour markers for BMPM.

10.4.1 Well-Differentiated Papillary Peritoneal Mesothelioma

Well-differentiated papillary peritoneal mesothelioma (WDPPM) is an uncommon subtype of epithelioid mesothelioma [19]. WDPPM, very rare, appears in the peritoneum of young women but may also present itself in the lining of the pleura. WDPPM rarely involves the testicular tunica vaginalis [20]. The clinical and imaging features of WDPPM are given in Table 10.1 [9].

This type of mesothelioma is defined as benign, but it may develop into a malignant form of mesothelioma. A new classification system proposed by Brimo et al. [20] has allowed stratification of mesothelioma into three categories: (1) well-differentiated papillary mesothelioma (WPDM), (2) mesothelioma of uncertain malignant potential, and (3) malignant mesothelioma.

The pathogenesis of WDPMP is poorly understood. Occasionally, asbestos exposure has been associated with development WDPPM [21]. Both malign such as gynaecologic renal, colorectal, pancreatic, and breast cancers and benign diseases such as adenomyosis, ovarian serous cystadenoma, mucinous cystadenoma, and teratoma have been proposed in the development of WDPPM [22]. However, there is no definitive etiologic factor that has been confirmed with reliable studies yet. WDPPM may occur in combination with other rare type of benign mesotheliomas such as BMPM and benign adenomatoid mesothelioma [23].

10.5   Diagnosis

Although WDPMP is usually seen in young women, it can occur in age ranges from 2 to 74 years [21]. WDPMP can present with acute and chronic abdominal pain, weight loss, chronic pelvic inflammatory disease, and ascites [19]. However, WDPMP is frequently asymptomatic and often an incidental finding during surgery or a radiologic examination for other reasons. WDPPM has rarely been described in the radiology literature due to the lack of specific radiologic features. The size of WDPPM tumour nodules ranges from 0.5 cm to several centimeters in diameter. WDPPM may present with plaque calcification that diffusely involves the visceral and parietal peritoneum without the presence of a significant associated soft tissue mass [24].

10.6   Pathology

WDPPM is characterized by uniform, coarse, or branching papillae covered by a single layer of mesothelial cells with only slight cellular atypia (Fig. 10.9a). Cystic areas were lined by papillary and tubulopapillary structures (Fig. 10.9b).

There is no gold standard immunohistochemical panel to cover all the diagnostic "mesothelial cells originated pathologies". The International Mesothelioma Panel recommends at least two mesothelial markers and two markers for the other tumour (dependent on the differential diagnosis based on morphology) besides a pancytokeratin. Tumour cells can be positive for D240 and anti-mesothelin (Fig. 10.9c). The Ki-67 index might be low in WDPPM (Fig. 10.9d).

10.7   Management of WDPPM

Most WDPPM have been reported to behave in a benign or indolent fashion, and death due to WDPMP is highly unusual [25]. However, WDPMP should be considered as a low-malignant potential due to tumour recurrence and occasional malignant transformation after resection of primary tumour. These findings support the designation of WDPPM as a low-grade tumour [26, 27].

Management of WDPMP still remains controversial. Patient outcome is usually favourable after tumour debulking surgery, without adjuvant therapy.

In Hoekstra et al. [27] series, 7 out of 38 cases with WDPPM died during follow-up although two of them were unrelated to the disease.

However, after complete tumour debulking surgery, the patient can show a recurrence on short-term follow-up [19]. Adjuvant therapy can be successfully a treat-

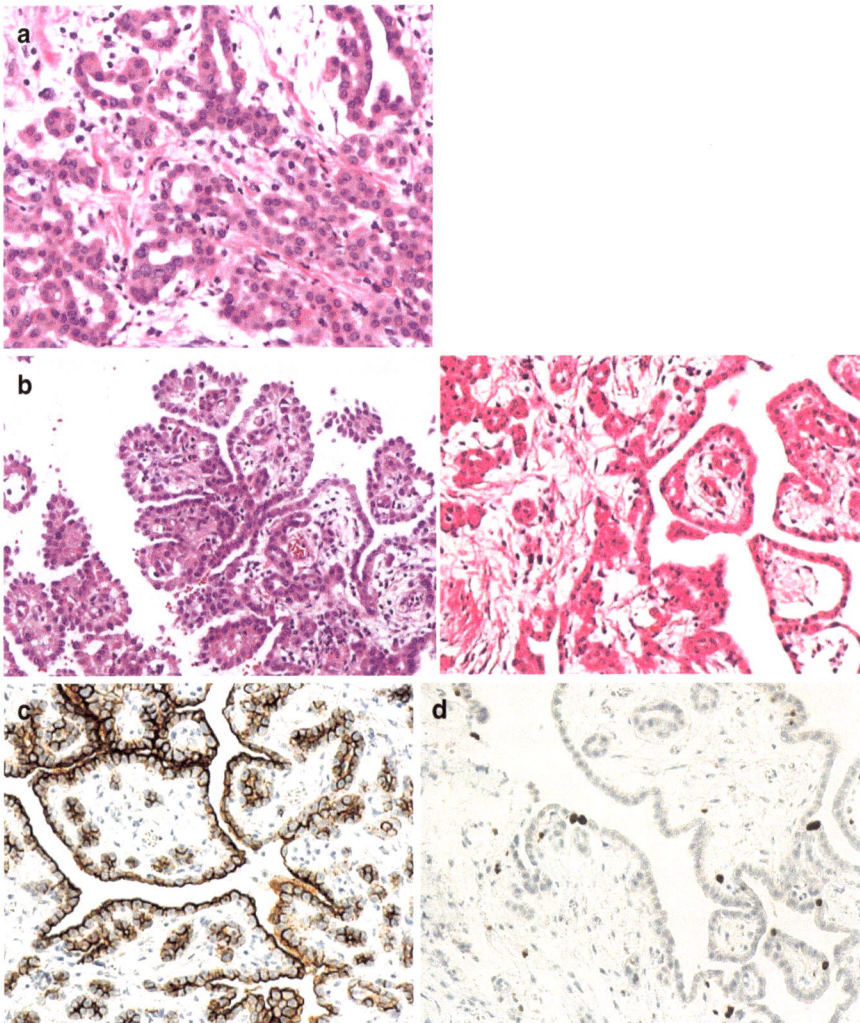

Fig. 10.9 (**a**) Papillary mesothelioma tumour shows numerous papillary, tubulopapillary, and spheroid/glomeruloid structures arranged in a *solid* pattern with few inflammatory cells (H&E, ×100). Papillary mesothelioma. (**b**) Cystic area is lined with distinct papillary and tubulopapillary structures and filled with foamy macrophages and lymphocytes (H&E, ×100). (**c**) The tumour cells are positive for mesothelin (×100). (**d**) Ki-67 staining of WDPPM

ment of choice in these cases. Close observation or serial biopsy for surveillance of WDPMP is necessary for early recognition of possible recurrences and malignant transformation [25]. Few cases of WDPPM progressed to epithelial type of diffuse malignant peritoneal mesothelioma (DMPM) [26, 28].

High recurrence rates and transformation into truly malignant and potentially lethal mesothelioma of DMPPM have been reported supporting the rationale of an aggressive approach with CRS and HIPEC.

There is only one series of DMPPM treated with aggressive surgery followed by heated intraperitoneal chemotherapy (HIPEC) [18]. In this report, eight cases of BMPM were reviewed by Baratti et al. [18]. Disease control was achieved in all patients treated with cytoreductive surgery with HIPEC except one patient who died of disease progression due to transformation into malignant biphasic mesothelioma.

They concluded that WDPPM is capable of transformation into invasive and potentially lethal process. Therefore, the definition of low-malignant potential tumours seems more appropriate to describe their nature.

In our experience (unpublished data), we have three patients with BMPM. We have performed complete cytoreductive surgery and HIPEC to these patients. So far, none of them had a recurrence or malignant transformation.

These results suggest that cytoreductive surgery to remove all visible tumour and heated intraoperative intraperitoneal chemotherapy to control microscopic residual disease will help patients with BMPM to remain disease-free and to obtain long-term overall survival.

Based on these findings, definitive tumour eradication with complete cytoreduction with peritonectomy procedures and HIPEC seems to be the optimal treatment to prevent either disease progression and recurrence or transformation to aggressive type of mesothelioma.

10.7.1 Benign Adenomatoid Mesothelioma

Benign adenomatoid mesotheliomas (BAMs) are benign rare tumours primarily found in the genital tract organs [29]. BAM can also develop in extra-genital sites including the heart, pleura, mediastinum, adrenal, intestinal mesentery, and omentum [30]. The clinical and imaging features of BAM are given in Table 10.1 [9].

Because these tumours are benign and usually diagnosed incidentally, there has been some controversy regarding the histologic origin of these tumours, but recent evidence has supported a mesothelial origin [30]. BAM are benign diseases, and therefore surgical excision of the tumours is both diagnostic and therapeutic, without the need for further intervention. None have ever been observed to recur or undergo malignant degeneration [29]. Therefore, there is no need to consider aggressive surgery and HIPEC in this type of benign tumours originated from mesothelial cells.

10.8 Conclusion

Benign multicystic mesothelioma and well-differentiated papillary peritoneal mesothelioma may have recur and transform malignant form of mesothelioma. An aggressive surgical approach with complete disease eradication is the goal of treatment.

From worldwide experience, cytoreductive surgery to remove all visible tumour and heated intraoperative intraperitoneal chemotherapy to control microscopic residual disease will help patients with benign multicystic peritoneal mesothelioma and well-differentiated papillary peritoneal mesothelioma to remain disease-free with a single surgical intervention. Disease eradication may prevent recurrence and transformation to an aggressive and fatal disease process.

References

1. Canbay E, Yonemura Y. "Peritoneal surface malignancies: a curative approach" book Chapter 3. Springer and Switzerland.
2. Momeni M, Pereira E, Grigoryan G, Zakashansky K. Multicystic benign cystic mesothelioma presenting as a pelvic mass. Case Rep Obstet Gynecol. 2014;2014:852583.
3. González-Moreno S, Yan H, Alcorn KW, Sugarbaker PH. Malignant transformation of "benign" cystic mesothelioma of the peritoneum. J Surg Oncol. 2002;79(4):243–51.
4. Iacoponi S, Calleja J, Hernandez G, Sainz dela Cuesta R. Asymptomatic peritoneal carcinomatosis originating from benign cystic peritoneal mesothelioma. Ecancer Med Sci. 2015;9:605.
5. Weiss SW, Tavassoli FA. Multicystic mesothelioma. An analysis of pathologic findings and biologic behavior in 37 cases. Am J Surg Pathol. 1988;12:737–46.
6. Ross MJ, Welch WR, Scully RE. Multilocular peritoneal inclusion cysts (so-called cystic mesotheliomas). Cancer. 1989;64(6):1336–46.
7. Mennemeyer R, Smith M. Multicystic peritoneal mesothelioma: a case report with electron microscopy of a case mimicking intra-abdominal cystic hygroma (lymphangioma). Cancer. 1979;44:692–8.
8. Gonzalez-Moreno S, Yan H, Alcorn KW, Sugarbaker PH. Malignant transformation of "benign" cystic mesothelioma of the peritoneum. J Surg Oncol. 2002;79:243–51.
9. Park JY, Kim KW, Kwon HJ, Park MS, Kwon GY, Jun SY, Yu ES. Peritoneal mesothelioma: clinicopathologic features, CT findings and differential diagnosis. Am J. 2008;191:814–25.
10. Villaschi S, Autelitano F, Santeusanio G, Balistreri P. Cystic mesothelioma of the peritoneum. A report of three cases. Am J Clin Pathol. 1990;94(6):758–6.
11. Safioleas MC, Constantinos K, Michael S, Konstantinos G, Constantinos S, Alkiviadis K. Benign multicystic peritoneal mesothelioma: a case report and review of the literature. World J Gastroenterol. 2006;12:5739–42.
12. Canbay E, Ishibashi H, Sako S, Kitai T, Nishino E, Yonemura Y. Late recurrence of benign multicystic peritoneal mesothelioma complicated with an incisional hernia. Case Rep Surg. 2013;2013:903795.
13. Pinto V, Rossi AC, Fiore MG, D'Addario V, Cicinelli E. Laparoscopic diagnosis and treatment of pelvic benign multicystic mesothelioma associated with high CA19.9 serum concentration. J Minim Invasive Gynecol. 2010;17:252–4.
14. O'neil JD, Ros PR, Storm BL, Buck JL, Wilkinson EJ. Cystic mesothelioma of the peritoneum. Radiology. 1989;170:333–7.
15. Soreide JA, Soreide K, Korner H, Soiland H, Greve OJ, Gudlaugsson E. Benign peritoneal cystic mesothelioma. World J Surg. 2006;20:560–6.
16. Van Ruth S, Bronkhorst MWGA, van Coevorden F, Zoetmulder FAN. Peritoneal cystic mesothelioma: a case report and review of the literature. Eur J Surg Oncol. 2002;28:192–5.
17. Sethna K, Mohamed F, Marchettini P, Elias D, Sugarbaker PH. Peritoneal cystic mesothelioma: a case series. Tumori. 2003;89(1):31–5.
18. Baratti D, Kusamura S, Nonaka D, Oliva GD, Laterza B, Deraco M. Multicystic and well-differentiated papillary peritoneal mesothelioma treated by surgical cytoreduction and hyperthermic intra-periotneal chemotherapy (HIPEC). Ann Surg Oncol. 2007;14(10):2790–7.

19. Nasit JG, Dhruva G. Well-differentiated papillary mesothelioma of the peritoneum: a diagnostic dilemma on fine-needle aspiration cytology. Am J Clin Pathol. 2014;142(2):233–42.
20. Brimo F, Illei PB, Epstein JI. Mesothelioma of the tunica vaginalis: a series of eight cases with uncertain malignant potential. Mod Pathol. 2010;23(8):1165–72.
21. Daya D, McCaughey WT. Well-differentiated papillary mesothelioma of the peritoneum: a clinicopathologic study of 22 cases. Cancer. 1990;65:292–6.
22. Rathi V, Hyde S, Newman M. Well-differentiated papillary mesothelioma in association with endometrial carcinoma: a case report. Acta Cytol. 2010;54:793–7.
23. Chen X, Sheng W, Wang J. Well-differentiated papillary mesothelioma: a clinicopathological and immunohistochemical study of 18 cases with additional observation. Histopathology. 2013;62:805–13.
24. Lovell FA, Cranston PE. Well differentiated papillary mesothelioma of the peritoneum. AJR. 1990;155:1245–6.
25. Malpica A, Sant'Ambrogio S, Deavers MT, Silva EG. Well-differentiated papillary mesothelioma of the female peritoneum: a clinicopathologic study of 26 cases. Am J Surg Pathol. 2012;36(1):117–27.
26. Burrig KF, Pfitzer P, Hort W. Well-differentiated papillary mesothelioma of the peritoneum: a borderline mesothelioma-report of two cases and review of literature. Virchows Arch A Pathol Anat Histopathol. 1990;417:443–7.
27. Hoekstra AV, Riben MW, Frumovitz M, Liu J, Ramirez PT. Well differentiated papillary mesothelioma of the peritoneum: a pathological analysis and review of the literature. Gynecol Oncol. 2005;98:161–7.
28. Hejmadi R, Ganesan R, Kamal NG. Malignant transformation of a well differentiated peritoneal papillary mesothelioma. Acta Cytol. 2003;47:517–8.
29. Schwartz EJ, Longacre TA. Adenomatoid tumours of the female and male genital tracts express WT1. Int J Gynecol Pathol. 2004;23:123–8.
30. Delahunt B, Eble JN, King D. Immunohistochemical evidence for mesothelial origin of paratesticular adenomatoid tumour. Histopathology. 2000;36:109–15.

Index

© Springer International Publishing AG 2017   137
E. Canbay (ed.), *Unusual Cases in Peritoneal Surface Malignancies*,
DOI 10.1007/978-3-319-51523-6